The Ultimate Body

By Liz Neporent

The Ultimate Body

Weight Training for Dummies

Fitness for Dummies

Fitness Walking for Dummies

Abs of Steel

Buns of Steel: Total-Body Workout

The Ultimate Body

10 PERFECT WORKOUTS FOR WOMEN

LIZ NEPORENT, M.A.

BALLANTINE BOOKS • New York

A Ballantine Book
Published by The Ballantine Publishing Group

Text copyright © 2003 by Liz Neporent, M.A.
Foreword copyright © 2003 by Ken Germano
Photographs copyright © 2003 by James Jankiewicz

Library of Congress Control Number: 2002096123
ISBN 0-345-45373-5

Text design by Helene Berinsky
Cover design by Carl D. Galian
Cover photo © Jim Cummins/Getty Images

Manufactured in the United States of America

First Edition: January 2003

10 9 8 7 6 5 4 3 2 1

For Jay . . .

I'll love you always.

CONTENTS

ACKNOWLEDGMENTS

If it weren't for the ten models who patiently gave their time and energy to pose for the pictures in this book, I honestly don't think my message that "fitness is possible for everyone" would have come through as clear as I hope it has. None of these women are professional models—though one has some part-time modeling experience—and, as you can see, they come in all different shapes and sizes. Yet, all possess a self-confident radiance that comes from being fit and healthy. They're living proof that looking and feeling your best is an achievable goal for all women. For this, I thank them.

Thanks to James Jankiewicz for taking the pictures and to Alison Rand and Gabe Walsh for letting me work in their apartment till all hours of the night and for teaching me way more than I ever wanted to know about Adobe Photoshop! I also need to thank my editor, Maureen O'Neal, for her expert guidance through the book-writing process.

My extreme appreciation goes to Ken Germano, Cedric Bryant, and the entire American Council on Exercise organization for their support for this book and for their relentless quest to improve professional standards in the fitness industry.

Many thanks to my Plus One Fitness business partners, Mike Motta, Bill Horne, and Jay Shafran, as well as the entire Plus One team, especially my partners "in crime," Grace De Simone, Bob Welter, John Buzzerio, Michele

Bibbey, Todd Crevistan, Courtney Farmer, Nancy Ngai, and Neal Pire. I learn from all of you every day.

To my parents, sister, brothers, nieces, nephews, and all of my in-laws— thanks for your encouragement. Ditto to my good friends Patty Buttenheim, Norman Zinker, Stephen Harris, Mary Duffy, Jackie Gardner, and Suzanne Schlosberg. With everything that went on this year, I couldn't have made it without you. There will always be a special place in my heart for Melissa McNeese and her family, as well as Alex Ham and Diane Naitztat for their emotional support and for giving us a place to stay post–September 11.

Thanks to my longtime readers who have followed all of my books, articles, and appearances. You are what makes writing about health and fitness such a rewarding and worthwhile experience. I invite you to post all of your questions and comments to my "Fit by Friday" message board located on www.iVillage.com.

And last but never least, I don't have the words to express how grateful I am for my husband, Jay Shafran, who is without a doubt the most supportive person on the face of the earth.

FOREWORD

We live in a world of fast, faster, fastest. Everything we do, everything we touch, every product we use or consume is supposed to get us there faster or produce a faster result. As a society we have been conditioned by savvy marketers and infomerchants to think and act in this speedy manner. That's probably why we so readily pour our hard-earned resources into anything we think will help us get something done quickly.

This is especially true when it comes to fitness. We're suckers for anything that promises to help us immediately shape up, transform our bodies, or drop weight. We're seduced by guarantees of instant fitness success, especially if it seems to require absolutely no effort on our part. We spend billions of dollars a year on diet books and cheap, flimsy exercise equipment.

And then we are absolutely amazed when our wallets are the only things that grow thinner.

Now that more than sixty percent of the population is considered either overweight or obese, diabetes is epidemic, and the incidence of heart disease is at an all-time high, it's time to question our get-fit-quick mentality and start getting serious about getting in shape the healthy way, the correct way—the permanent way.

This is why I am pleased to recommend the information and exercise routines in *The Ultimate Body*.

In this book, Liz Neporent leads you simply and logically through the development of your very own personal exercise foundation. She understands that everyone's foundation is unique and that you must take an individual approach to fitness if you want to succeed.

On a daily basis we are bombarded with information regarding exercise and weight loss. Most of it is inaccurate and or based on someone's biased, uneducated opinion. It's so disappointing to watch that so-called experts with zero credentials making millions of dollars selling products that inevitably wind up as coat racks in your home or PennySaver ads. By following the programs found in *The Ultimate Body*, you'll make some major strides toward leaving all of this misguided, misdirected misinformation behind and achieving your new or renewed personal fitness goals.

Liz Neporent is a degreed, certified, and time-proven expert. She has spent half her life helping people develop successful, long-lasting exercise habits. She understands the basic tenets of fitness, exercise, and physical activity as they pertain to daily living and achieving your fitness goals and dreams.

The Ultimate Body is compiled of surefire methods for success when it comes to building your path for life long physical conditioning. Liz's expertise is supported by industry experts, user testimonials, and a compendium of highly respected and credible resources. This volume is one of the most complete and comprehensive guides to better fitness and physical wellbeing that I have seen in my thirty years in the fitness industry.

You only have one you, and you've made the right choice in selecting *The Ultimate Body* to help yourself get in shape. What are you waiting for? Get started on your "Ultimate Body" today. In fact, invite a friend, your wife, husband, children, mother, or father and get them started on their "Ultimate Body," too.

Good luck on your road to lifelong fitness!

Ken Germano, M.A.
Executive Director
The American Council on Exercise
www.acefitness.org

The
Ultimate
Body

HOW TO USE THIS BOOK

Welcome to *The Ultimate Body: Ten Perfect Workouts for Women*. You're here to find out the answers to questions like "What is the absolute best way to sculpt my butt?" or "How do I flatten my abs?" or "How can I stay in shape while I'm traveling when I can't find a decent gym?" You've come to the right place for honest, accurate, realistic information about exercise and making positive body changes.

This book contains the very best information available on how to attack your most stubborn fitness problems. It's based on my twenty years of experience as a personal trainer and fitness expert as well as feedback from researchers, educators, and other respected authorities. You'll also hear from clients and readers—people just like you—about what's worked for them.

I can tell you this: It's all about exercising the right way for your goals on a consistent basis. It's the only guaranteed way I know to get results. And it really works.

Too often, people are unrealistic about what it takes to get in shape. It's not entirely their fault. We've been brainwashed into thinking that all you need to lose weight or reshape your thighs is some pill, powder, or potion. I know that every time I scan a magazine, the Internet, a book, or TV I'm bombarded with fitness misinformation. Just this morning I listened to an infomerchant scream into the camera about how you can transform your body to your exact specifications in less than six weeks without exercising or changing your eating habits. (All that's required is three easy payments, credit cards accepted.)

Can you make significant changes to your body in six weeks? Absolutely. In fact, I'm going to show you how to do it within the pages of this book. But can you do it without exercising and eating right? Of course not. This is something we'd all like to believe but know is too good to be true.

Look, in a moment of desperation or frustration, who hasn't bought a gadget that promises to melt away fat from your abs or spot-reduce your thighs? This book will help you stop wasting your time, energy, and megabucks on get-fit-quick schemes and start focusing on the reality: If you want to get in shape and change your body, you're going to have to do something about it.

I'm not saying you have to kill yourself to get the body you want. Far from it. This book will teach you to work smarter, not harder. And I promise you that if you follow my advice, you will make significant improvements to your body, your fitness level, and your life.

"My original fitness goal was to lose about ten to fifteen pounds," remembers Patty, a forty-two-year-old poultry farmer from Virginia. "I had tried many times to take off some weight, and I think the main reason I hadn't had success was that I wasn't doing any exercise." As soon as she began exercising, Patty not only succeeded in reaching her original goals, she exceeded them. She dropped three dress sizes and feels more confident, more energetic. But the best part, she claims, is that she no longer has to obsess about what she eats or worry about the number on the scale. "It's amazing how much this has carried over into my daily living," she says.

I get letters and comments like that all the time. The principles in this book have helped many of the women I've worked with do things like lose over a hundred pounds, realize their dreams of doing a triathlon, and tighten up the jiggle in the backs of their arms. I know these same principles can help you achieve great results, too.

And I promise you that all of the programs in this book are straightforward and easy to follow. You can do them. I've carefully put together the most effective moves possible into ten perfect workouts. They're designed to achieve targeted results quickly; you won't have to dedicate hours a day to working out. I'm a firm believer in making your workouts fit into your life and not the other way around.

I know you're chomping at the bit to get started on your workouts, and I'm glad you're here. But I do want you to take some time to understand what this book is all about and how you can use it to your best advantage.

How to Use This Book

There are ten chapters devoted to specific workouts. All of them are designed to sculpt and tone a particular muscle group or body area or help you solve a specific fitness problem. I've selected all of the exercises in each chapter because they are the most effective, results-oriented moves you can do. They're also safe and unlikely to cause any injuries.

Depending on what your goals are, you can use just one of the chapters as your main workout, add the routine in a chapter to a workout program you're already doing, or mix and match several workouts to address multiple fitness concerns. The workouts can also be used in combination. Let me give you a brief overview of each chapter and how best to use each of them.

- **The Perfect Beginner Workout:** This workout contains everything a beginning exerciser needs to do to get started working out. If you have never exercised or it's been at least six months since you've taken a single step or moved a muscle, I suggest starting with this workout. It gives you a six-week workout progression to follow and slowly builds you up from doing nothing to becoming a full-fledged exerciser. I recommend using this as a stand-alone workout for at least six weeks; after that you can consider combining it with the other workouts in this book to target individual areas. However, you can always use the Perfect Stretch Workout as a warm-up or the Perfect Mind-Body Workout as a cool-down.

- **The Perfect Weight Loss Workout:** This chapter contains tips on successful weight loss based on scientific research, the personal experiences of my readers and clients, and good old-fashioned common sense. I give you a fast-paced circuit workout, which is a sort of hybrid of aerobics and strength training. It's designed to burn calories and pump up your resting metabolism by building muscle. I think this is best used as a stand-alone workout. However, you can alternate the Perfect Weight Loss Workout with one of the area-targeted programs, such as the Perfect Leg and Butt Workout or the Perfect Abdominal Workout, if your goal is to lose weight and reshape a specific part of your body. But remember, you'll lose weight more quickly if you focus the majority of your efforts on this workout, which is designed explicitly to help you drop pounds. You can use the Perfect Stretch Workout as a warm-up or the Perfect Mind-Body Workout as a cool-down if you have the time and if they don't distract you from putting your energy into your primary goal—losing weight.

- **The Perfect Upper-Body Workout, the Perfect Leg and Butt Workout, and the Perfect Abdominal Workout:** All three of these chapters will zero in on a single zone of your body and sculpt it to perfection. The exercises in each of these chapters are designed to give you results even if an area has not responded well to exercise in the past. Although you can use any of these chapters as a stand-alone workout, I think they work best when they're folded into a total body routine. You can do them all on the same day or rotate through them on separate days.

- **The Perfect Strength Workout:** The exercises in this chapter are classic strength-building moves. This is the perfect workout for you if you are looking to build pure strength and/or muscle size. It works well as a stand-alone routine or when you alternate it with the Perfect Mind-Body Workout for a nicely balanced, hard/easy program.

- **The Perfect Gym Workout:** If you work out at a gym and have no clue how to use the equipment, the workout in this chapter is the perfect solution. It's a full-body workout that makes the most of exercise equipment—especially the weight-training equipment—your gym is likely to own. If you don't always work out in the gym, then alternate this with a combination of the Perfect Upper-Body Workout, the Perfect Leg and Butt Workout, and the Perfect Abdominal Workout or the Perfect Travel Workout. You can also alternate it with the Perfect Mind-Body Workout if you want a program that balances cardio and muscle building with flexibility and stress reduction.

- **The Perfect Stretch Workout:** I like to use this workout as a warm-up for the routines in the other chapters or at the end of any workout as a cool-down. Use this workout as a stand-alone chapter if your aim is purely to improve flexibility.

- **The Perfect Mind-Body Workout:** This gentle workout is the very best routine to promote calmness, reduce stress, and increase flexibility. You can alternate it with any of the other routines as a way to balance out more-strenuous workouts. It can be used as a stretch workout at the end of any of the other routines as well.

- **The Perfect Travel Workout:** Because you don't always have access to exercise equipment when you're on the road, I've included a cardio/strength-training workout that does not require any fancy equipment. Use it when you travel or if you work out at home and don't have any exercise paraphernalia at your disposal.

Workout Descriptions

The workout chapters all follow a similar format to make them easier for you to use. At the beginning of each workout chapter, you'll find a brief description about the information contained within the chapter as well as a list of all the equipment you need to do the routine.

All of the exercise descriptions are set up approximately the same way. They include any information you need to know about the exercises and how to do them correctly. This is the format they follow:

- **Muscles Worked:** This section lists the main muscles targeted by the exercise. Typically I list the muscle that is the "prime mover" first, followed by all of the "assister" muscles in size order from largest to smallest.

- **Joint Cautions:** Just because I give a joint caution for an exercise does not mean it is dangerous or unsafe. I've chosen the exercises in this book not only for their effectiveness but also because they carry a relatively low risk. A joint caution simply means that if you have issues with the joint or muscles listed, you should pay extra attention to make sure that the move causes no pain or discomfort. Most of the time, the exercise will actually help reduce problems in the weakened area by strengthening the specific muscle in question and all of the surrounding muscles. However, any exercise that causes sharp, pinpointed pain should be avoided. If you have major problems with a particular joint or muscle, I suggest you try the easiest version of the exercise first and see how it goes.

- **Starting Position:** Technique is the most important aspect of any exercise—it's more important than how many reps or sets you do or how much weight you lift. If you just look at the photo of each exercise without reading the text, you'll miss valuable pointers on how to do the exercise correctly. Obviously, starting in the correct position is the key to doing an exercise correctly.

- **Exercise:** It bears repeating: Good technique is the most essential aspect of any exercise. In this section, I tell you everything you need to know to do the movement correctly.

- **Things to Think About:** In this section I tell you exactly where you should feel the exercise; this will help you determine whether or not you are doing the exercise correctly. Sometimes I relate the movement to something else to help give you a mental picture of what you should look like when performing the exercise. I also give you some important reminders about correct technique and give you a heads-up on some common ways you can go astray. I've trained a lot of people using these exercises, so I have a pretty good idea about what form reminders you'll need.

- **Variations:** For almost every exercise in this book I give you at least one variation that's more challenging than the basic version and at least one that's less challenging. This gives you a lot of flexibility. If the basic version doesn't feel right or it's just a little beyond you right now, you can drop down to the easier variation. As you progress and you're ready for more, you can move on to the harder version.

Fit-tionary

Almost any organized activity has its own vocabulary. Skateboarders have their Misty Flips and Nose Grabs, wine aficionados have their bouquets and tannins, medical doctors have their *Helicobacter pylori* bacterium and depressor labii inferioris ligaments. Exercise is no different. There is a common vocabulary that helps you better understand what you're doing every time you pick up a weight or tie the laces on your walking shoes. Fortunately, it's an easy language to learn.

Below I've defined some terms I use frequently throughout this book. I'm sure you'll also hear them bandied about by other people who are into exercise. I'll give you reminders about these definitions here and there as you move through subsequent chapters, but I thought it would be useful to give you some in-depth explanations and put them all in one place so you can see how they relate to one another.

BASIC TERMS

Cardiovascular: This refers to any activity you do with the purpose of strengthening your heart and lungs and burning calories. It's also known as cardio or aerobic exercise. In order for a workout to be considered cardiovascular, it has to involve large muscle groups used in a continuous, rhythmic fashion and last for more than a few minutes. Running, walking, cycling, and swimming are the most popular forms of pure cardio exercise.

Strength: Theoretically strength is defined as the maximum amount of weight you can lift one time, but that's not typically how most of us use the term. We think of strength as how much weight a muscle can lift or how much work it can do over the course of about a minute. In scientific terms this is known as muscular endurance, but for simplicity's sake, let's stick to the word *strength!*

Flexibility: How far and easily you can move your muscles is known as flexibility. Flexibility varies from joint to joint, muscle to muscle. You improve flexibility by stretching your muscles on a regular basis.

Workout: Sometimes called a routine or workout routine, a workout is one exercise session. There are ten workouts in this book, all designed to bring about a specific result. Ideally, all workouts should be designed to achieve a specific goal.

Program: When you take a step back and look at how all of your workouts fit together in a daily, weekly, and monthly pattern, you are viewing your entire exercise program. It's not a bad idea to take a global look at your program on a regular basis; this will help you determine whether what you're doing is working well or whether it needs some tweaking. It also helps you plan your future workouts.

Warm-up: Every workout in this book includes a recommendation for a warm-up or is a warm-up in and of itself. Doing a five-to-ten-minute warm-up at the start of every workout is essential to raise your body temperature, increase blood flow to your working muscles, and increase muscle pliability. All of these things help prepare your body to work harder, perform better, and prevent injury.

Cool-down: The workouts also include a recommendation for a five-to-ten-minute cool-down at the end of every workout so your body doesn't just do an instant shift from exercising to rest. This is a defense against injury and also prevents you from sweating through your clothes even after you've showered.

WEIGHT-TRAINING TERMS

Weight Training: The term "weight training" has several synonyms—"weight lifting," "resistance training," "strength training," and "body sculpting." Actually, the term "weight training" is somewhat of a misnomer. You don't have to lift a weight to build muscles and reshape your body. Anything that places more stress (or resistance) on your muscles than they normally encounter will help build, sculpt, and strengthen. Besides dumbbells, barbells, and weight machines, special exercise bands made of strong rubber tubing can also provide resistance. Even your own body can be used as a "weight." When you do any of the squat exercises in this book that call for you to bend down into a sitting position, you probably won't need any additional weight for the first few weeks of your exercise program, as pushing your body weight against gravity will be plenty challenging enough.

Weights: Weights come in all shapes and sizes. Barbells, for instance, are long metal bars with weighted discs attached at either end; sometimes these discs are removable and interchangeable, and sometimes they're permanently locked into place. Dumbbells are short metal bars. They're similar to barbells except you hold one in each hand rather than with both hands. Weight machines are large contraptions that usually consist of a weight stack and a series of levers, cables, and pulleys. The weight machines you find at most gyms are generally used for no more than one or two exercises, whereas the weight machines you buy for home allow you to do multiple exercises.

Though there are certainly differences between free weights and machines, and between gym machines and home machines, I think they all do a good job of working your muscles provided you use excellent form and work out on a consistent basis. You may find you have a preference for a particular kind of weight training. I say whatever way is the most comfortable and enjoyable is the right way to train.

Exercise: Also known as *move*. This is the movement you take your body through to achieve a specific result.

Repetition: Sometimes referred to as *rep* for short. A repetition is one complete movement of an exercise, such as when you bend and straighten your arm to do a biceps curl.

Set: A set is a one complete group of repetitions. For example, when you do fifteen push-ups in a row, that equals one set.

Rest: *Rest* refers to the amount of rest you take between sets and the amount of rest you take between workouts. The rest you take between sets usually ranges from zero to about ninety seconds. You take this rest so your muscles have time to recover and "reset" themselves, giving your body a chance to give its best effort on all subsequent sets. The rest you take between workouts allows your muscles to repair themselves from the tearing-down process of weight training. For adequate rest, muscles need at least forty-eight hours between workouts. However, you can still weight-train every day so long as you don't lift with the same muscles two days in a row. You might want to work your legs one day and then follow that with an upper-body workout the next.

Breathing: I make a bigger deal about breathing in some chapters than in others. I used to make a really big deal about breathing all the time, but I found that many of my clients just got confused about when they should breathe, how they should breathe, and where they should be breathing from. The simple answer is this: When doing weight training and active stretch exercises, exhale through your mouth as you exert an effort and inhale through your nose as you release an effort. For any move that calls for holding one position for a long moment, just keep breathing deeply in and out for as long as you hold the position.

Can't keep this straight? Don't worry about it. A lot of people get frustrated when they can't remember these rules. Unless you're doing heavy duty power lifting or hoisting tree trunks over your head in one movement, the important thing is to just keep breathing!

CARDIOVASCULAR AND FLEXIBILITY TERMS

Maximum Heart Rate: The fastest your heart can beat is known as your maximum heart rate; it's measured in number of beats per minute, or bpm. To estimate your maximum heart rate, subtract your age from 220. (Studies show that at its peak, the human heart can beat about 220 times per minute, and this maximum seems to decline by about one beat per minute every year after age twenty.) Keep in mind this is an estimate at best. Your maximum heart rate can vary up or down from the age-based prediction by as many as fifteen beats, depending upon heredity, general health, and overall fitness. Your true maximum heart rate can be determined by going to a doctor and having a stress test; it can also be more closely estimated by a skilled and experienced trainer via a bike or treadmill evaluation.

Target Heart Zone: Also known as your target training zone or THZ, your target heart zone is the range of acceptable heart rates your heart should beat while exercising. Your THZ is a percentage of your maximum heart rate; most experts think that for safety and best results, you should exercise at between 50 and 90 percent of your max. If you base these numbers upon your age-predicted max they may be off. To determine your range of exercise heart rates, multiply your max by .5 and .9. Of course, that's a pretty big range. In later chapters I will talk more about when to be at the top of your range versus the bottom.

Intervals: Interval training calls for you to alternate spurts of exercise done at the low end of your training range with spurts of exercise done at the high end. This is a great way to experiment with faster speeds and higher intensities without having to commit a whole workout to pushing yourself to the limit. It also makes things more interesting than doing the same thing for an entire workout.

Range of Motion: This is a flexibility term that refers to how far you can move a joint. So, for instance, if you can bend over and touch your toes with no problem, that is your hamstrings' range of motion. If you can't touch your toes, your hamstrings have a restricted or limited range of motion.

PERFECT MOTIVATION

On September 11, 2001, the senseless terrorist attacks on the World Trade Center and the Pentagon changed all of our lives forever. For me, the changes were more immediate than for most. I live and work about half a block away from the World Trade Center site in New York City and was in the epicenter of this terrible, tragic event as it unfolded.

Although my home was uninhabitable for a period of time and my livelihood was significantly affected, I consider myself one of the lucky ones: I narrowly escaped with my life as the towers collapsed around me, ultimately walking out of the destruction without so much as a scratch. Everyone I love and care about who was also in the area (including my husband) is alive and well.

I know this seems like a funny way to start a chapter on getting motivated to exercise, but this experience opened my eyes about what it means to lack the motivation to move. I want to share what I've learned with you so that you know you're not alone if you sometimes have trouble getting started. Almost everyone at some point or another needs a push to get going.

To tell you the truth, I never really understood why it is so hard for people to get into exercise. For me, working out has always been as natural as breathing. I mean, why sit on the couch watching *Simpsons* reruns and eating Doritos when you could be out exploring a new running route, scrambling up rocks, or pumping iron in the gym with a couple of friends?

But after September 11, for the first time in my life I was too sad and depressed to move a muscle. I could barely walk my dog around the block, let alone lift a weight or run a step. I knew from experience and education (and from telling other people to do it) that getting some exercise would make me feel better, but I just couldn't bring myself to begin.

After a couple of weeks of complete inactivity, I had a long talk with myself. I agreed to do a little something every day, even if it was just to go for a quick walk or do a few moments of stretching. In the past, I'd always exercised to keep my weight under control, to shape my body, or for competition, but now I needed exercise to give me the strength to deal with everything I was going through.

I didn't dive back into my usual routine, which is probably hard-core by most people's standards, but I didn't let myself completely off the hook, either. I gave myself permission to ease into a scaled-down version of what I typically do, just to get myself back in the game. And you know what? It did help me cope. It helped me a lot. The more I did, the better I felt, so the more I was able to do. After a few weeks I was back to my old exercising self.

This experience taught me a couple of important lessons. First of all, sometimes pushing yourself to work out is really hard. I know this is probably an obvious conclusion to the more than 80 percent of Americans who don't work out on a regular basis, but it wasn't to me. This revelation has helped me relate much better to my clients and readers.

Second of all, there are many different reasons why people aren't motivated to exercise. You have to address each of these reasons head-on in order to overcome them. That's what I'd like to do in this chapter.

Being in the business of getting people into shape for as long as I have, I've noticed that most people have roughly the same excuses for not exercising. I'm not saying these "exer-scuses" aren't valid or that they're always easily dispensed with—but you *can* conquer them. I'd like to address the most common antiexercise objections with you now and give you some solid strategies for getting your butt in gear.

Excuse #1: I Don't Have Enough Time

Between carpooling the kids, dropping off the dry cleaning, and staying late at work to finish up a project, it seems as if there are never enough hours in the day for everything you need to do, let alone exercise. And in fact, most people claim they don't exercise due to a poverty of time. A recent *Ladies' Home Journal* poll found that more than 35 percent of women cite lack of time as their number one reason for not exercising or eating well, and a recent Fitness Products Council poll found that nearly 75 percent of Americans age thirty to forty-four would like to work out more often but can't find the time. I could tick off similar results from dozens of other polls, surveys, and studies, but I think the point is made.

Time management is a problem for all of us, but I often find that the busiest people are the ones who are avid exercisers. So how do these sweat-loving high achievers fit fitness into their lives?

- **Prioritize.** "I couldn't find the time until I found the time, if you know what I mean," says Jan, a thirty-two-year-old executive assistant. I think that's true. If you've ever gone through a period where you did exercise consistently, you probably weren't any busier than you are right now. "If getting into shape is truly something you feel you have to do, then you somehow find a way to get it done. I can't explain how it works, but it's as if time suddenly appears in your day," Jan theorizes. Jan also admits she struggles to get to the gym when she goes through extremely busy periods in her life. When that happens she shortens her workouts rather than skipping them altogether. "Frequently, the only difference between when you exercise regularly and when you don't is that you've made it one of your priorities," she says.

- **Schedule.** Violet Zaki, one of my favorite exercise video stars, once told me that when it comes to working out, she does what she says she's going to do, not just what she feels like doing. That comment has always stuck with me. I think about it every time I feel like skipping a workout I have planned.

  Write down your workout appointment or zap it into your Palm Pilot. Then when the time comes, keep that appointment with yourself as if you are the most important client in the world. (You are.) Bottom-line it for yourself. If you decide that it's important to you to achieve the body of your dreams, exercise becomes a can't-miss proposition.

- **Seize opportunities.** I always tell my clients to keep spare workout gear on hand in case the opportunity presents itself to exercise. Sometimes a meeting is canceled or your mom pops in and offers some impromptu baby-sitting—what a waste to have a block of time if you don't have your walking shoes! Keep your gear in your briefcase, your pocketbook, the backseat of your car, or any other place that's usually accessible—you might catch a lucky break.

- **Work out smarter, not longer.** Unless you're training for the Olympics or a marathon, you don't need to dedicate your entire life to working out. When it comes to exercise, the more-is-better mentality really doesn't apply. The trick is to figure out what your goals are and then do just enough to achieve them. That's what the workouts in this book are designed to do. Most can be done in under an hour; some take far less time than that.

- **Break it up.** Still don't think you have enough time? It's not necessary to do all your exercise at once. Studies show it's just as effective to do a little here, a little there. For instance, doing a ten-minute walk in the morning, a ten-minute walk at lunch, and a ten-minute walk in the evening will give you the same results as one half-hour walk. To create the time you need for this particular workout, you might get up ten minutes earlier, go to bed ten minutes later, and shorten your lunch break by ten minutes.

Excuse #2: It's Too Hard

I once heard a comedian say that he'd tried lifting weights but they were too heavy. I think many people have that same impression, that exercise is very, very hard. This is partially the fault of those of us in the fitness business. We push too many workouts that are beyond what someone just starting out is capable of doing; we cater to the 20 percent of people who are already in good shape and leave everyone else out in the cold.

That's not to say that you won't have to put in the work or that exercise doesn't sometimes cause discomfort. I would be doing you a disservice if I withheld the truth about that. But exercise does not have to be an awful, painful, miserable experience. I promise you, it can be quite enjoyable, especially when you get past the first few weeks, the period of time where you're most likely to struggle and experience some aches and pains. In the workout chapters I give you tips and tactics for starting out at the appropriate level and gradually progressing into a more challenging routine. Here are some other commonsense guidelines to help you avoid most of the discomfort.

- **Ease into it.** You *cannot* make up for years of slothfulness with one workout. This is one of the most common mistakes new exercisers make. If you do a ninety-minute, all-out barn burner of a workout your first time out, guess what? It's going to be hard. You're going to wake up the next day so sore that lifting your coffee cup to your lips will be a challenge. You won't exactly be inspired to continue. Take it slow to start. If you're unable to complete one of the workouts, no worries. Do what you can and build from there.

- **Listen to your body.** It really does know best. If it's telling you you're exercising too hard, then you're exercising too hard. You're more likely to hurt yourself if you push past your comfort zone. Besides, going full tilt won't necessarily give you better results. Did you know you burn about 100 calories a mile whether you walk it or run it? So if a leisurely stroll is all you can handle without huffing and puffing, by all means slow things down a bit.

- **Gauge your intensity.** Everyone, but especially beginning exercisers, can benefit from gauging exercise intensity. Knowing when to push harder and when to back off can be somewhat of an acquired skill; having some tangible method of measuring intensity helps you accurately determine how your body is responding to exercise. These are the three most common ways to measure workout intensity.

- **Heart rate.** How fast your heart beats corresponds directly with how hard you're exercising. The more intense the exercise, the faster your heart beats.

  You're not looking to hit an exact heart rate each time you work out, but rather somewhere within a range. This range is called your target heart zone. Your target heart zone is the range of heart rates within which your heart should be beating for a given intensity of exercise. It is based on your maximum heart rate, or the fastest your heart is able to beat under any circumstances. Estimate your maximum heart rate is by subtracting your age from 220. Then multiply this number by .5 and .9 to come up with your target heart zone. Beginners should do the majority of their workouts toward the lower end of the range. This will help avoid soreness and injury. After a few weeks you can begin to explore the upper regions of your target heart rate zone.

  During your workout, you can take your heart rate, or pulse, at your wrist or your neck. To do so, place your index and middle fingers lightly on the vein located at the base of your thumb or at the groove at the side of your neck; count the number of beats you feel in fifteen seconds, then multiply by 4. If you're no mathematician, count the beats you feel in ten seconds and add a zero. Check your heart rate after you've been working out for at least five minutes.

  If all this poking, prodding, and multiplying is too complicated for you, consider purchasing a heart rate monitor. This device comes with a strap that wraps around the bottom of your chest; it transmits an accurate heart rate to a large wristwatch or to the display on most cardio machines found in the gym. I like Polar heart rate monitors the best; they're reliable and, at around $50 to start, reasonably priced.

- **RPE.** Rated perceived exertion (RPE) is a 1–10 scale that helps you measure how hard you're exercising. It saves you the trouble of taking your pulse in the middle of a workout. Simply pay attention to how your muscles feel, how much you're sweating, the sound of your breathing, and anything else that contributes to your feeling of exertion, then assign a number corresponding to your total overall effort. On this scale, 1 is very, very easy and 10 is a near all-out effort.

- **Talk test.** Here's how the talk test works: During your workout you should be able to carry on a breathless conversation. If you can trip along singing "The Thong Song" at the top of your lungs, you need to speed up. If you can't form the words "Sweet fancy Moses, this is hard work," then you need to slow things down.

Excuse #3: It's Boring

You may have the idea that exercise is boring, but when you actually do it you may discover that that isn't the case. Repetitive activities such as walking and jogging don't require much concentration and may help you into a more relaxed, calmer mental state similar to that found in traditional meditation, a state of mind that many experts feel is ideal for creative thinking, problem solving, and easing stress.

On the other hand, you may find that exercise is as stimulating as, say, watching paint dry. If so, you've probably asked yourself more than once, "Isn't there any way to make this stuff more exciting?" Yes, there is.

- **Cross-train.** Doing the same exercise routine day after day is like eating the same thing for every meal, points out Cynthia Kereluk, star of Lifetime cable's *Everyday Workout.* "That would get pretty monotonous after a while and make it almost impossible to get all the nutrients you need." Exercise isn't much different. Alternating several fitness activities is a practice known as cross training. You might consider doing different workouts in this book to help prevent boredom and overemphasizing one aspect of training over another.

- **Get creative.** Walking and running are great activities, but some people find them mind-numbingly boring. Luckily, anything that raises your heart rate and keeps you moving will exercise your body. I have a group of clients who are avid Ping-Pong players. That might not seem like much of anything, but it's a sport that requires stamina, strength, coordination, and agility. They get their heart rates up and have a good time.

- **Distract yourself.** If you walk into any of the gyms that Plus One (the company I work for) designs, you'll notice TVs in front of every piece of cardio equipment, music playing on the loudspeakers, and signs advertising CD players and radios for loan. That's because most people like to have some distraction while they work out, to make the time go faster. If watching TV or listening to your favorite tunes floats your boat and keeps you moving longer, I say crank up the volume. Just be careful about getting too distracted if you're exercising alone in a deserted area or someplace where there is heavy traffic.

- **Find a buddy.** If you're tired of your own company, try exercising with a partner. Choose someone who's supportive, responsible, and likes the same activities you do. You can also join a club or put together an informal group as well. Debra, one of my iVillagers and a homemaker from Washington State, likes working out with a group and has allowed this concept to grow with her program. She started out with a walking group, and when she lost interest in walking she began taking kickboxing classes. She recently joined a Jazzercise group. I applaud her creativity and willingness to adapt.

Excuse # 4: I Don't See Results

Admit it. After a killer set of abdominals, it's tempting to run to the mirror to see if your stomach looks any flatter. Of course, it probably doesn't. As anyone who's ever begun an exercise program knows, you can't expect to see a complete metamorphosis overnight.

Many people abandon their exercise programs when they don't see results as quickly as they'd like. A *Ladies' Home Journal* poll of over three thousand women found that feeling frustrated from lack of results was the number two reason they abandoned their exercise programs (lack of time was the number one reason).

I can tell you that if you stick with it, you *will* see results. How long it takes depends on a lot of things, including where you're starting from, genetics, how dedicated you are to your workout schedule, your age, and a list of other factors. While you're waiting, these strategies should help.

- **Be realistic.** You didn't get out of shape in one day, so don't expect to snap back into shape overnight. But at the same time, keep the faith that it will work. Sandra, a forty-two-year-old marketing manager from Chicago, admits that not being able to believe that her program would work after so many failed attempts kept her from trying again for a long time. "But I stuck with it even when I didn't see much happening for the first few months," she says. Now that she's lost eighty-five pounds, she's glad she did.

- **Set goals.** You want to lose weight, but how much? For example, you would ideally like to weigh what you weighed in high school (fifty pounds lighter), but your doctor says it would be a good start if you would just take off ten pounds. What you aim for doesn't have to be your final goal, but it will help you get focused. The more specific, the better. In order to set goals, you should have a good idea where you're starting from. It's smart to jot down your current weight or percentage of body fat so that you have something to check it against later on. At iVillage we do a roll call every Monday that asks for your starting weight, current weight, and goal weight.

- **Track progress.** How do you know if you are accomplishing what you set out to do? By keeping a training log so you can see where your improvements and weaknesses are. A simple calendar or weekly planner will do.

- **Use your failures.** "I guess you could say I have failed at my previous workout programs," says Jonathan, a Portland, Oregon, student. "I remember once I used a weight-lifting routine that was too intense for me; I ended up overtraining and not making any gains. But really, it wasn't a failure, because I learned more about myself and my body. After I failed at a workout program that was probably for someone on steroids, I learned that my body could not take that much intensity. So I made a mental note and moved on from there." I think Jonathan has a great perspective. The road to success is often paved with a few failures along the way. As the marines say, "Fall down seven times but get up eight."

Excuse #5: I'm Too Self-Conscious

Do you walk past mirrors and avert your eyes? Margie used to. "I could not stand the way my body looked, so I stopped looking, I went something like two years without seeing my body," she admits.

Margie also admits that she didn't want anyone else to see her body, either, and that's what kept her from working out. She couldn't stand the thought of walking into a gym or going for a walk outside; she felt like everyone was looking at the cottage cheese on her thighs or the roundness of her belly. Here's what she and others like her do to get past that feeling of self-consciousness.

- **Find support.** A lot of my clients and readers tell me that support is the number one thing that has helped them achieve their fitness goals. So enlist your husband, coworkers, kids, friends, gardener—anyone you know will be a good cheerleader for you. You may choose to work out with a buddy or organized group; hiring a personal trainer may also be a good idea.

- **Find your place.** If you're just too self-conscious to work out in public, then home workouts will probably be best for you, at least to begin with. But keep in mind that there are all different kinds of gyms and support groups out there. Curves for Women caters to women who need to lose weight; a place like that might offer much-needed support, more than you'd get by exercising at home by yourself. There are also gyms that cater to bodybuilders, runners, rock climbers, busy executives, and just about any other group you can think of. You may find motivation by being in an environment where you're surrounded by people with similar goals.

- **People are self-involved.** Entering a gym for the first time can feel a lot like being the new kid at school. You think people are checking you out and passing judgment. Trust me, for the most part this isn't true. People are somewhat narcissistic by nature, and while they may look up when you first walk through the doors or pass by, they usually return to looking at themselves pretty quickly. They're almost always more concerned with how they look and what they're doing than they are with you—they don't have the time, energy, or interest to pay attention to you.

PERFECT QUESTIONS,
PERFECT ANSWERS

Between my iVillage message boards, my clients, and the people who read my books and articles, I often get asked over five hundred fitness-related questions a week. At this point, I believe I've been asked just about every possible question there is about fitness, exercise, and getting into shape. "What is the best workout for my hairstyle?" "Is the pogo stick a good cardiovascular activity?" And once, I swear, "How many calories does childbirth burn?"

I told the woman who wanted to know about the best workout hairstyle to get a haircut, the pogo stick fancier that bouncing up and down on a metal pole can deliver a decent workout provided you can stay on long enough, and the mother-to-be who was concerned with fat burning while giving birth to reconsider her priorities. (I really have no idea how many calories you burn during labor and seriously doubt that science has bothered to measure such a thing.)

I try to answer every query sent my way as accurately and honestly as possible. Not all of them are weird and wacky. In fact, I find the majority of people want to know about the same basic issues, more or less.

In this chapter, I've sifted through the thousands of questions I've received over the years and pared them down to the ten most frequently asked. I bet you've been searching for the answers to some if not all of these. I will continue to remind you about a lot of this information in other chapters, but I think this is an excellent place to set the record straight on some major issues.

What Is the Best Aerobic Exercise?

The aerobic workout you will actually do is the best aerobic exercise for you. That's the workout you're most likely to stick with long enough and work at hard enough for it to make changes to your body.

Studies show that when people are allowed to choose their most comfortable pace, they tend to burn the most calories on a treadmill compared to a bike, aerobic rider, ski machine, rowing ergometer, or elliptical trainer. The bike and aerobic rider machines tend to be the slowest calorie burners.

But what if you think of the treadmill as a dreadmill? How long are you likely to trudge along before you bail due to sheer boredom? And if you enjoy pushing the pedals on your cycle or bucking back and forth on your aerobic rider machine, you're more likely to extend your workout and thus burn more calories as well as give your heart, lungs, and muscles a more thorough workout.

So the trick is to find something you actually like to do. Don't like to walk? Then run, hop, skip, jump, hike, climb, kickbox, skate, ski, or swim. If you like company when you exercise, take classes, join a running club, or find a workout partner. If you're competitive by nature, enter some road races, take up a sport that keeps score (such as tennis, racquetball, or golf), or track your personal bests and try to beat them. If you're easily bored, watch TV while you sweat, hire a trainer, or alternate among a whole array of different activities. With so many choices, you are bound to find something you can at least tolerate.

I truly feel that most people who say they hate to exercise simply haven't searched hard enough for the right activity. I was serious when I said that jumping on a pogo stick is an effective way to get in shape. It hits virtually every muscle in your body, burns about 650 calories per hour, and does a decent job upping heart rate—though fear of crashing into the bushes probably accounts for at least some of the increase in heart rate.

Any activity that you can sustain for five minutes or more; that uses the larger muscles of the legs, arms, or torso in a rhythmic fashion; and that gets your heart pumping will give you the aerobic benefits of burning calories and strengthening your cardiovascular system. To be truly effective, the activity must keep your heart beating in its target zone nearly the entire time; for most people that's between 60 and 90 percent of maximum heart rate. (For more on target heart zone, maximum heart rate, and how to determine them, see chapter 1.)

Will Certain Aerobic Workouts Bulk Up My Thighs?

I don't know why a few irresponsible fitness-product informerchants tell women that healthy activities such as running and stair climbing will blow their legs up to the size of redwoods, but I do know this theory is utterly false. This pervasive myth makes me really angry, because if you buy into this nonsense, it narrows your exercise choices unnecessarily. Here is the real scoop.

It's not the specific cardio activity in and of itself that makes your thighs bigger—it's the way you do your cardio. Any aerobic-type activity done slowly and using a heavy resistance will bulk up your lower body. It's pushing against a lot of tension, like the heavy gear on a bike or a harder level on the stair climber, that creates larger, chunkier muscles. If you aerobicize using light resistance and move at a faster speed, you're far less likely to bulk up.

Of course, some women *are* more susceptible to building larger thighs no matter what they do. This is a simple fact of genetics. I myself have very muscular legs. But so does every other woman in my family, even the ones who don't exercise as much as they should. If your legs tend to gain muscle easily, stick to light-resistance cardio training; for instance, on a bike, spin at a high rpm on a lighter gear, or on a treadmill, do speed walking rather than slow uphill climbs.

Won't Lifting Weights Give Me Big, Bulky Muscles?

This is another pervasive myth that won't die. The fact is, unless you spend hours and hours in the gym lifting impossibly heavy weights, it's unlikely you will build the large, chunky muscles you see on bodybuilders and power lifters. Most women don't have enough of the male hormone, testosterone, coursing through their veins to build gargantuan amounts of muscle.

I think some women fear bulking up because they leave too much to the imagination. They think they're going to get bigger, so they feel bigger. I get a lot of feedback from women who swear to me that their thighs or butts have swelled to mammoth proportions after a couple of weeks of lifting moderate weights twice a week. When I ask for before-and-after measurements, most women haven't taken them, so they don't really know whether they've gained size or not. If you don't keep accurate measurements, you're just guessing.

Women who are mesomorphs, a body type characterized by a solid build with hips and shoulders that are approximately the same width, may tend to add muscle more easily than other body types, though even a mesomorph will probably not be able to pack on mountains of muscle. However, mesomorphs may build enough muscle to make their clothes feel slightly tighter, especially if they don't lose fat as they gain muscle.

If you are a mesomorph and making your tailor rich is not one of your goals, you will have to be sure to include enough cardiovascular activity in your fitness program to keep your body fat down as you add some extra, healthy muscle onto your frame. This extra calorie burn should solve your clothing dilemma.

With consistent workouts mesomorphs tend to sculpt and shape well-defined muscles more easily than the slender, underwear-modeling ectomorph body type or the curvy, voluptuous endomorph body type.

Rather than trying to escape your shape, why not embrace it? Why not train it to be the best it can be? All body types look better with regular weight training. Madonna is a famous example of a buffed-up mesomorph. So are Sarah Jessica Parker and Gloria Estefan. Michelle Phillips, Ashley Judd, and Jennifer Love Hewitt are classically fit ectomorphs.

Cindy Crawford, Jennifer Lopez, and Britney Spears are excellent examples of well-toned endomorphs. Now, do any of these women look too bulky to you?

Which Are Better, Free Weights or Machines?

Using free weights (bars and dumbbells) allows you to be more creative and flexible with your weight-training program. You can literally do hundreds of exercises with only two or three sets of dumbbells. Add a bench, some extra weight plates, and maybe a few different-shaped bars and you have enough equipment to work out for a lifetime without breaking the bank.

Some experts do think that free weights work the muscles more efficiently than weight-training machines because they require a high degree of balance and skill to use; this means you use many of the smaller, deeper muscles that otherwise would get a free ride. However, because you need all the balance and skill, free weights can be challenging to master. There is a learning curve for every new exercise you add to your repertoire. Free weights are also potentially dangerous, especially if you don't take the time to learn proper form or if you stop paying attention. I have seen broken feet, smashed dental work, and bruised ribs—all a result of careless dumbbell handling.

Beginning in the 1960s, machines have been designed with a distinct advantage over free weights: They are fitted with a special pulley, called a cam, that varies the amount of weight you lift during each phase of the exercise. So if you are doing a biceps curl, for instance, the weight feels lighter at the start of the movement, where you are weakest, and heaviest at the top of the movement, where you have the best mechanical advantage. When you do that same exercise using free weights, you are limited to the weight you can manage in the weakest part of the movement.

Strength-training machines also have the advantage of being safe and easy to use. Typically they are designed for one or two exercises, so their levers move in only a finite number of ways; this makes them much easier to learn and use. They allow you to fly through your workout more quickly because you only need to make a few simple adjustments before doing an exercise.

There's a down side to machines as well. They're expensive and take up a lot of space. Plus they only allow you to do one or two movements. I know I said this was an advantage, but it is also a disadvantage. Because you can do only a few exercises on each machine, you need a lot of them. Ultimately workouts lack variety and begin to feel stagnant and boring.

So which type of weight-lifting equipment is the better choice? I say both are good. I personally believe that you get the best results when you combine the two, using free weights for some exercises and machines for others. The trick is to experiment and find out which way of mixing and matching suits you and which gives you the best results.

Will This Supplement Help Me Lose Weight Faster?

It seems there is always some new diet supplement that claims to help you lose weight without exercise or careful eating. As I write this, science has yet to discover any supplement that makes a significant, *safe* contribution to weight loss. I think we will have effective weight loss aids in the future; there is some interesting research going on in the field, but it will probably be decades before scientifically proven weight loss supplements will be available to the public.

But for now, the truth doesn't seem to matter. New supplements are introduced weekly, and Americans keep spending billions of dollars on these pills, powders, and potions. Supplement manufacturers get rich, and the only thing that gets thinner is our wallets.

Why do we fall for false promises and bogus claims every time? Because the marketing is so seductive. Let me give you a classic example.

Infomerical products that promise instant and dramatic weight loss are certainly nothing new. But when a product claims to take the place of exercise and allow users to eat as much as they want without gaining an ounce, it's bound to raise a few eyebrows. That was precisely the premise of Enforma Natural Products' infomercial for their Exercise in a Bottle and Fat Trapper supplements.

In the half-hour program, former baseball player Steve Garvey and nutritionist Kendall Carson told viewers they could consume high-calorie foods and still lose weight simply by taking a few pills with every meal. Exercise in a Bottle's active ingredient, pyruvate, purported to work by "forcing every cell in your body to work harder whether you're exercising or not." Fat Trapper was a combination of chitin, a fiber derived from shellfish, and chitosome, a plant fiber they claimed "literally traps fat before it gets into your system."

To bolster the claims of pyruvate's influence on weight loss, the infomercial quoted a University of Pittsburgh study, which found that subjects who took supplements of the substance had a 48 percent greater rate of fat loss and 38 percent greater rate of weight loss than those who didn't use pyruvate.

Here's the kicker: This information was absolutely on the level. If you looked up the study, you would find that it was accurately reported. However, when you take a closer look at the evidence, you begin to see how even credible research can be presented in a misleading way.

The study looked at obese, bedridden women on 1,000-calorie-a-day diets—hardly normal circumstances for most dieters. Though the percentages of fat loss and weight loss are quoted correctly, the subjects who took the pyruvate lost only 3.52 pounds more than those who didn't—far less than the significant losses implied by the infomercial. Researchers also gave the women in the study thirty-six grams of pyruvate daily—about ten times the recommended dosage of Exercise in a Bottle.

To prove the effectiveness of chitin and chitosome, Garvey poured bacon grease into a glass of water. Because globs of fat formed and fell to the bottom when the contents of four Fat Trapper pills were added, he declared this proof of Fat Trapper's ability to absorb up to 120 grams of fat.

The Fat Trapper demonstration was a gross distortion of science. The aforementioned study took a grain of truth and spun it into a desert. In reality, chitin and chitosome only bind fat to a small degree. They absorb 3–5 grams—the equivalent of a pat of butter. The few human trials performed on chitin and chitosome have pronounced them ineffective as weight loss aids. For instance, two Italian studies found they contribute a small additional weight loss *when combined with a low-calorie diet*. Some researchers speculate that long-term use of the supplements might lead to nutritional deficiencies because they may prevent the body from absorbing fat-soluble substances such as vitamin D, vitamin E, and essential fatty acids.

Consumer groups were so outraged by Enforma's claims, they sued the company for false advertising. The FDA finally stepped in and fined Enforma more than $10 million for making bogus claims and using misleading statements in their ads. But Enforma made hundreds of millions of dollars on the products before they were finally pulled from the market in early 2000.

We cannot always count on government agencies to protect us from these supplement schemes. There are too many supplement scams and too many loopholes in the laws. At best, these supplements are ineffective; at worst, they can have serious, long-lasting side effects. Consumers need to resist false promises. If it sounds to good to be true . . . well, you know the rest.

I've Recently Lost Weight. What Can I Do About Loose, Flabby Skin?

Fat that builds up around your trouble spots causes your skin to stretch out in those places. But when you lose a significant amount of weight, you are likely to notice some looser-looking skin in those areas. Your skin is elastic, but once stretched out, it does not completely spring back into shape.

How readily your skin tightens up after a big weight loss, if at all, depends largely upon genetics, how long you were heavy, and your age (the younger you are, the better the chance of no permanent bagging and sagging).

Women who have lost a significant amount of weight tell me that common trouble zones include an "apron" around the waist, the sides and fronts of the knees, and the backs of the upper arms. Although skin in and of itself does not respond to weight training, the muscles underneath these areas probably will to some extent. This is yet another reason why you should weight-train as part of your weight loss efforts and continue even after you've reached your goals.

I almost never recommend cosmetic surgery, since it is such a deeply personal choice, but in the case of excess skin, this may be an option worth considering. This is especially true if you've lost several hundred pounds, as some of my clients have; often after such a dramatic weight loss, you can be left with twenty-five to fifty pounds of excess skin. Most surgeons will not perform this type of operation until you've kept the weight off for at least a year. If you do decide to take this route, research it carefully.

How Much Exercise Do I Really Need?

Probably not as much as you think if your goal is disease prevention and building moderate amounts of strength and stamina. According to the American College of Sports Medicine, a respected scientific organization that makes health recommendations to the public, all this requires is about twenty minutes of cardio activity three to five times a week, about twenty minutes of strength training twice a week, and a few minutes of daily stretching. The surgeon general's office makes it even easier for you: It recommends thirty minutes of moderate activity nearly every day; this activity can include everything from conventional exercise to gardening to walking to the corner store for a quart of milk, and it doesn't have to be all at one time.

However, if your goals are serious weight loss or body sculpting, you need to make a bigger commitment to exercise. But even then it's all about working smarter, not spending more time in the gym. I discuss in detail exactly what you need to do to achieve those goals in the workout chapters

What Is the Best Way to Lose Weight?

High-protein diets, my personal least-favorite diet fad, allow you to eat greasy burgers and fat-marbled steaks provided you abstain from bread, potatoes, rice, and other carbohydrates. Many people do lose weight on this sort of plan. (In fact, many recent studies show that high-protein diets may help you lose weight faster than low-fat diets in the short term and with fewer ill effects than we once thought. There are no studies that I know of that have examined long-term success or detrimental health hazards of eating high protein. If it turns out I'm wrong about high-protein diets in the future, I'll happily admit it.) Then, after a few weeks of carnivorous eating, this is what usually happens: Their taste buds grow weary of eating the same things day after day, so they begin slipping more carbs back into their diets. Inevitably the pounds begin to pile on again.

What amazes me most about this scenario is that people blame themselves for the failure, not the diet plan. They come away with the belief that carbs are the culprit and that if they just had more willpower, they would have succeeded. They never stop to think that their weight gain is due to the fact that *they began eating more total calories.*

The tried-and-true formula for losing weight—eat less, move more—is incredibly simple, yet the majority of people don't seem to believe it works. Most people pursue weight loss by starving themselves, following fad diets, buying expensive weight-loss products, or trying some other quick-fix weight loss scheme. Ironically, they turn to sensible eating and regular exercise only out of desperation.

I think part of the problem is that people want instant gratification. They want to see a total transformation overnight. Weight loss marketing is designed to play into this get-fit-quick mentality. There's a $30 billion diet industry counting on it.

Another part of the problem, I think, is that people are asking the wrong question. They ask "How do I lose weight?" when they should be asking "How do I lose weight and *keep it off?*" Almost any of the diet products available will help you lose weight, including those ubiquitous high-protein plans—*but only in the short term.*

Maybe because exercise and eating well don't come with an outlandish claim or a quirky gimmick, people don't believe they will get results. Perhaps it's because they bring about results more slowly in the short term than quick-fix weight loss methods. I don't know what to tell you except that a combination of workouts and healthy eating is the one proven method that actually does what it promises. For a detailed account on this, flip to "The Perfect Weight Loss Workout," chapter 4.

How Quickly Will I See Results?

This is a question I wish I had a definitive answer for, but I can only say this: It depends. It depends upon how much effort you put into your workout routine. It depends on how seriously you overhaul your eating habits. It depends upon your genetics. And, of course, it depends on what results you are looking for.

I've carefully designed each of the workouts to give you results in the quickest, safest way possible. I've laid out a section in each of the workout chapters giving you approximate estimates of how quickly you'll see results from doing the routine as recommended. I also tell you about what results you can expect at various points in time. But please keep in mind I'm giving you *estimates:* You may see improvement more quickly or slowly, depending on the factors I named above. Please don't beat yourself up if you don't see results as quickly as my estimates predict—or as quickly as you'd like.

Beware any product or program that claims to deliver the goods in a definite amount of time. There is just no way to predict your body's response. We are all individuals and progress at our own individual rates. The key is consistency and patience. Though each workout brings you one step closer to where you want to be, don't expect one or two workouts to bring about a total overhaul. One thing I can guarantee you, though—you stick with it, you *will* see results.

What's the Best Exercise to Flatten Abs?

Or trim thighs? Or reduce saddlebags? Or make a bust look bigger? Let me bottom-line it for you: You cannot spot-reduce an area—that is, melt fat off a specific part of your body—by exercising it. The body simply does not work that way. We all have individual genetic profiles that dictate where, when, and how we lose weight. If you are highly prone to retaining a spare tire of fat around your middle, no abdominal exercise in the world will give you chiseled, washboard abs without some weight loss.

You can, however, lose weight by watching what you eat and making exercise an integral part of your life. Along with that, you can spot-tone and spot-change areas on your body with targeted weight-training exercises. That's what this book is all about.

THE PERFECT
BEGINNER WORKOUT

Working with overweight women who were just starting an exercise program gave Grace, a certified personal trainer, a whole new perspective on the exercise experience. "Most people work out to look a certain way, but these women had goals like pouring a glass of milk without straining their wrists or getting on and off the floor without assistance," she says. She admires the courage and discipline it takes to start from scratch and says her best advice is to increase slowly, do what you can even if you can't do it all, and be patient about getting results. The birth of her two children gave her further insight into the process of shaping up. "It's hard at first, and you do experience a little discomfort along the way, but once you begin to see and feel success—even a little bit—you'll be hooked."

EXERCISES IN THIS CHAPTER
- Kneeling Leg Press
- Modified Push-ups
- Pelvic Tilt
- Back Sweep
- Half Squats
- Toe Raises
- Shoulder Press

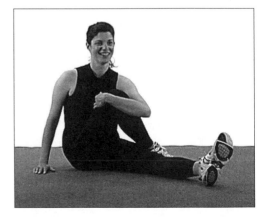

- Basic Biceps Curls
- Basic Triceps Dips
- Partial Ab Roll-up

EQUIPMENT NEEDED
- Two or three sets of light dumbbells
- A sturdy, stable chair or workout bench

ESTIMATED WORKOUT TIME
- First week: 30 minutes, three times a week;
  50 minutes, two times a week
- Second week: 30 minutes, three times a week;
  50 minutes, two times a week
- Third week: 40 minutes, three times a week;
  60 minutes, two times a week
- Fourth week: 45 minutes, three times a week;
  65 minutes, two times a week
- Fifth week: 45 minutes, three times a week;
  65 minutes, two times a week
- Sixth week and beyond: 45 minutes, two times a week;
  65 minutes, three times a week

"Honestly, getting myself started was the hardest part of working out," says Cathy, a part-time retail saleswoman from Cincinnati. At her heaviest, Cathy tipped the scales at 230 pounds. She didn't exercise, and she overate when her emotions got the best of her. She began her weight loss program by taking a good, hard look at herself and accepting that it was time to make some changes.

Have you reached the same point as Cathy yet? If so, you've come to the right place. In this chapter I'm going to give you some general guidelines to get yourself started—but, more important, guidelines for sticking with it. I'm going to tell you what you absolutely should do to stay on track and what you need to avoid so you don't derail your efforts. I'll take you step by step through the nuts and bolts of a beginner workout so you know what you should be doing and what results you can expect.

Sound good? Then let's get started by reviewing the immutable laws of fitness.

The Five Golden Rules for Beginning Exercisers

Cathy echoes an attitude common among novice exercisers: "When you don't see results right away, you get discouraged and make up excuses not to continue." That's true. How many times have you begun a shape-up program with a vengeance only to give up on the third day because you hadn't dropped a dress size yet?

So rule number one for getting into shape is this: *It takes time.*

Cathy's been at it for about five months. She's lost twenty-one pounds but knows she isn't there yet. She's in it for the long haul. "I have not reached my weight goal at this point, but I know I will in time. I didn't gain this much weight overnight, and I know it will not leave overnight," she says. And she's right. A mere week's worth of workouts is simply not enough to undo a decade's worth of sitting on the couch and stuffing your face with McDonald's. If you think it can, you'll need to readjust your thinking before you start.

However, this brings me to rule number two: *If you're consistent and you keep at it, you will see results.* Exercising and eating right are no genie in a bottle, instantly granting your wishes. They're more like the erosion of a rock—slowly, gradually making a difference over an extended period of time.

Perhaps the biggest fitness mistake I see people make, particularly those who want to lose weight, is going for the quick fix, be it a fad diet, protein shake, starvation regimen, electrical stimulation gadget, or some other drop-ten-pounds-in-forty-eight-hours type of miracle. Many of these things do work—in the short term. As everyone knows, it's easy to lose a few pounds. It's another thing altogether to maintain weight loss. If you want to make permanent changes, slow and steady wins the race.

Rule number three of our immutable shape-up laws: *Set specific goals.* I always say that if you don't know where you're going, any road will take you there.

Goals should be as explicit and as detailed as you can make them. For instance, you can say to yourself, "Gee, I wish I looked better," and that can be one of your major fitness goals, but if you define what that means in terms of scale weight, body fat percentage, inches lost, or any other parameter you can measure with precision, you'll be better off. Having a goal that's measurable gives you a way to track progress—or lack of progress. It also tells you when you've reached your destination.

Choose your goals carefully. They should be realistic and attainable yet meaningful. The most motivating goals are personal and chosen because *you* want to achieve them, not because your mother thinks you should lose weight or all of your friends have signed up for the spring walkathon.

That brings me to rule number four: *Have a plan.* Now that you have a goal, how are you going to make it a reality? Too many people jump into an exercise routine without the slightest idea of how what they do relates to the results they'll get. They may attack the weight room for a couple of hours when all they really want to do is build a little strength and tone up. Or they may take up running even though it's boring and painful and they hate it. Or they decide to lose weight without rethinking their eating habits or rearranging their schedule to fit in a daily workout.

The things you need to consider when you're putting together your master shape-up plan include how much time you have to spend on exercise, what equipment you have available or how much money you have to spend getting access to equipment, the best time of day to work out, and the best location to do it in.

Let's talk about that time commitment for a minute.

The number one excuse people give me for not working out is that they don't have time. This is what Patty, a self-employed Virginia poultry farmer, has to say about this topic: "So many people tell me that I'm so lucky to have the time to work out. I don't have any more time than anyone else. I make it a priority because it *is!* Sometimes that means leaving the laundry and dishes undone or asking my husband and teenage son to fix their own meal. You have to be willing to make that time for yourself."

You have the time if you want to find it. When working out becomes a priority, suddenly, as if by magic, blocks of time open up in your day.

And don't underestimate the importance of making your workout fun and enjoyable. Try to choose an activity that you don't rate right up there with having your teeth pulled out and put back in again. You won't last long if you pick something you loathe. From walking to swimming to rock climbing, there are literally a thousand different ways to work out. Scout around. Try new things. If you find something (or several somethings) you love to do, you stand a much better chance of actually doing it.

Finally, our last immutable law of fitness: *Expect to fail sometimes*. I know that sounds counterintuitive, but it's an important concept to grasp. Accept the fact that you can't go for the rest of your life without eating chocolate. Or that you're going to blow off an occasional workout. Or that you may have to stop in the middle of a run because you just don't feel like it today. These things are going to happen.

The difference between succeeding and failing is that when you have these setbacks, you start right up again without missing a beat. Don't let a single misstep turn into a week or a month or even years of missteps.

For the same reason, it's always wise to keep a set of backup goals in your hip pocket. Recently a woman named Josey posted a message on my iVillage Fit by Friday message board complaining that she had not been able to do her regular workout because of an injury. She said the most discouraging part was that she finally had been getting into a regular routine and now had to give it up because of knee pain that came out of nowhere.

I told her to change course rather than abandon her program entirely. She needed to look at it as an opportunity to focus on other aspects of her program she was probably neglecting, such as flexibility and weight-lifting technique. Josey wrote me back, thanking me for the advice. She's going to try some new exercises and begin taking yoga. Good for her. She now knows she doesn't have to throw in the towel every time life tosses a new roadblock in her path.

Your Shape-up Plan

A good fitness plan has three main components: cardiovascular, strength, and flexibility. By exercising your heart and lungs with cardiovascular (aerobic) workouts, you'll strengthen them so they work more efficiently;

you'll also bolster your immunity against many diseases, feel more energized, increase stamina, and, yes, lose weight, too.

Strength training not only does what its name advertises (makes you stronger) but also tones up your body, protects you from injury, bolsters your confidence, and aids in weight loss by speeding up your metabolism.

Flexibility work limbers you up in order to balance how loose your muscles are versus how strong they are. Stretching is an effective way to better your posture, reduce stiffness, and help you move more easily and fluidly.

The rest of this chapter deals with the cardio and strength-training workouts you should be doing as a beginning exerciser. As I said at the start of this chapter, I'll take you through each workout step by step. For a detailed guide on flexibility training, flip to chapter 10, "The Perfect Stretch Workout."

Your Perfect Beginning Cardio Plan

So many of my clients and readers are skeptical about walking as a means of getting into shape. Some people have a hard time believing that an activity as simple as walking will do anything for them. In fact, there is a growing body of evidence that suggests walking may be the most effective weight loss and fitness program for the majority of exercisers. Here's why.

- Walking is safe and easy to do for nearly everyone, including older folks, pregnant women, and those who are very out of shape. Almost everyone can start out on—and continue—a fitness program with walking. This makes it one of the easiest workouts in the world to keep up with.

- You can lose weight by walking, and there is plenty of science to support this claim. For instance, a large study sponsored by the National Weight Control Registry found that more than 80 percent of long-term "losers" used walking as their primary form of exercise. The faster you walk and the more you weigh, the more calories you will burn. A 150-pound woman who walks 3.5 miles an hour for an hour a day can burn about 300 calories. If she walks five days a week and watches the fat and calories in her diet, she can lose as much as 18 pounds a year.

- Walking is adaptable. You don't need to walk for an hour straight to make your walking program effective and to achieve your goals. You can accumulate this hour over the course of a day, which means you can adapt your walking program to fit your lifestyle and schedule.

- Among the health improvements you'll see from doing a regular walking program: decreased blood pressure; an increase in HDL or "good" cholesterol (by up to 6 percent, according to one study performed at the Cooper Institute for Aerobic Research); prevention of heart disease, diabetes, and some forms of cancer; preservation of bone density and prevention of osteoporosis. Because it's a weight-bearing activity—it places stress on your bones—walking stimulates the growth of bone cells. In short, walking can help you live a longer, healthier life.

- There is no denying the emotional benefits of walking, either. Study after study has found that it helps counter depression and relieve stress. It refreshes the spirit, often giving you a break from your hectic life; it's a wonderful way to stop and smell the roses without actually having to stop!

- Because walking is low-impact—less than half the impact of running—there is little chance of injuring yourself. I think this is the key to its success. A low injury rate means fewer excuses to drop out. You may not go very fast, but because you don't often get hurt you can go far and go often.

This is just a snapshot of the things walking can do for you. It seems that nearly every day some new study, some new piece of evidence, is published extolling yet another of walking's virtues. Perhaps that's why sixty-seven million Americans log over 201 million miles a year.

The walking program I've outlined for you assumes you've been doing nothing for at least six months. It's a six-week schedule that starts out by getting you in the habit of walking and then building from there. You may not feel like you're doing very much at first, but trust me, you are. Developing a consistent walking habit is no small accomplishment. This routine is designed to ease you into walking, and exercise in general, without a lot of soreness or discomfort. It's also designed to be super-flexible to eliminate those pesky "I have no time" and "I can't fit it in" types of excuses.

You should start to see results in the form of weight loss and increased stamina after about three weeks. As time goes on and you gradually build up time and intensity, those results will come even faster. After the first six weeks, you can repeat weeks three to six or flip to one of the other chapters for a more advanced workout.

For best results, combine walking with two or three days a week of strength training and daily stretching (more about the rules of strength training later in this chapter).

WEEK ONE: WALKING ASSIGNMENT

Goal:

We're taking this first week to get into the habit of walking. Consequently, our emphasis is on getting out there—whether outdoors or on a treadmill—and doing it no matter what. Your goal is to accumulate a total of thirty minutes of walking time at least six days this week.

Notice I said *accumulate*. That means you don't have to do the entire thirty minutes at once. If you get tired or run out of time, simply split up your walking time into two or three sessions throughout the day. At this point, it's an accepted scientific fact that you'll burn exactly the same number of calories and get almost the same health benefits as doing the entire walking workout in one shot.

As you walk, don't worry about your speed, intensity, or even how many calories you're burning. (We'll focus on those things in the weeks to come.) Get your body used to the art of putting one foot in front of the other. Take note of how your body responds to walking: what your breathing sounds like, how much you sweat, how the muscles in your legs feel, how your body moves, how long it takes before you feel tired.

For those of you who are planning on doing your entire walk at one time and are looking for some structure and guidance, here's a sample workout to follow. You can do this same workout every workout.

Interval	Time	Intensity
Warm-up	5 minutes	50–60 percent of your maximum effort Suggested speed: 2.5–3.0 mph Suggested hill grade: 0 percent
Main workout	20 minutes	60–70 percent of your maximum effort Suggested speed: 3.0–3.8 mph Suggested hill grade: 0–2 percent
Cool-down	5 minutes	50–60 percent of your maximum effort Suggested speed: 2.5–3.0 mph Suggested hill grade: 0 percent
Total	**30 minutes**	

WEEK TWO: WALKING ASSIGNMENT

Goal:

This week we're going to work on your technique and add in some strengthening exercises. You're going to walk the same times and distances as last week, while concentrating on your Focus on Form walking checklist (see sidebar on page 63).

You're still not too concerned about speed or distance. At this point you're still in the process of making walking a healthy lifestyle habit. Perfecting your walking form will help you in the weeks to come by making it easier to pick up the pace and to walk for longer periods of time without getting tired or injured.

WEEK THREE: WALKING ASSIGNMENT

Goal:

Time to kick it up a notch. This week we increase the duration of our walks.

You're going to up your walking time to forty-five minutes a day and aim for at least six workouts a week. The same rules still apply: You don't have to do your entire walk in one workout. It's okay to split it up into two or even three walks in a day. For instance, you can do a quick fifteen minutes on the treadmill first thing in the morning—a great way to rev you up at the start of your day. You can then do a quick spin around the neighborhood during your lunch break and finish up with another fifteen minutes to walk off your dinner.

Don't forget to practice good technique as you walk; refer to the Focus on Form checklist I introduced last week if you need a refresher. Good walking form will serve you well by giving you the stamina you need to go the extra distance.

For those of you who are planning to do all of your walking in one session, here's a suggested workout format for you to follow. At this point I'm giving you some feedback on how many calories you're burning, but remember, that's only part of the picture. By walking on a regular basis, you're also building muscle and increasing your metabolism. A faster metabolism means you burn more calories all the time, even while you're at rest. You may also find that regular exercise helps reduce appetite.

Interval	Time	Intensity
Warm-up	5 minutes	50–60 percent of your maximum effort Suggested speed: 2.5–3.0 mph Suggested hill grade: 0 percent
Main workout	30 minutes	60–70 percent of your maximum effort Suggested speed: 3.0–3.8 mph Suggested hill grade: 0–2 percent
Cool-down	5 minutes	50–60 percent of your maximum effort Suggested speed: 2.5–3.0 mph Suggested hill grade: 0 percent
Total	**40 minutes**	

WEEK FOUR: WALKING ASSIGNMENT

Goal:

It's time to rev up your engines. This is the week we fulfill your need for speed. With three weeks of walking under your belt, it's time to up the ante a little bit.

The goal this week is to do two of your workouts at a faster walking pace. This is going to increase the distance you walk in a given amount of time, so you'll burn more calories without having to increase your workout duration. Walking faster builds muscle, too; that means you burn more calories even at rest simply because your metabolism is stoked.

All of your other workouts stay the same (including your strength-training sessions). Doing just two high-speed workouts to start gives your body time to adjust to the increased effort. You're less likely to get injured when you gradually add fast paces into your workout rather than turning everything up a notch all at once.

Remember, though, you still have the option of splitting up your walk routine into several mini-workouts. For those of you who want a complete workout to follow, the chart below illustrates one way you can structure a speed workout.

Interval	Time	Intensity
Warm-up	5 minutes	50–60 percent of your maximum effort Suggested speed: 2.5–3.0 mph Suggested hill grade: 0 percent
Speed interval I	15 minutes	70–80 percent of your maximum effort Suggested speed: 3.8–4.5 mph Suggested hill grade: 0–2 percent
Rest interval I	5 minutes	60–70 percent of your maximum effort Suggested speed: 3.0–3.8 mph Suggested hill grade: 0–2 percent

Interval	Time	Intensity
Speed interval II	15 minutes	70–80 percent of your maximum effort
		Suggested speed: 3.8–4.5 mph
		Suggested hill grade: 0–2 percent
Cool-down	5 minutes	50–60 percent of your maximum effort
		Suggested speed: 2.5–3.0 mph
		Suggested hill grade: 0 percent
Total	**45 minutes**	

WEEK FIVE: WALKING ASSIGNMENT

Goal:

Things should be looking up at this point. All the more reason to add some hills to your walking routine. Your assignment this week is to add one workout where you walk up hills or, on the treadmill, inclines. This is where you'll see all of that speed work and strength training you've done in the previous weeks start to pay off. You'll need that extra strength and stamina to chug up the inclines.

Walking upward and onward is a great way to burn additional calories and tone the muscles of your butt and thighs. It's a good way to burn calories without increasing speed. In fact, if you find you like walking hills better than picking up the pace, feel free to substitute at least one additional hill workout in place of one of your speed workouts this week.

Just another reminder—chopping up your walk into several sessions is still fine so long as you accumulate a total walking time of forty-five minutes each day for six days this week. Below is a sample hill workout that you can try on the treadmill or outside.

Interval	Time	Intensity
Warm-up	5 minutes	50–60 percent of your maximum effort Suggested speed: 2.5–3.0 mph Suggested hill grade: 0 percent
Hill	3 minutes	75–85 percent of your maximum effort Suggested speed: 3.0–3.5 mph Suggested hill grade: 4–8 percent
Rest	2 minutes	60–70 percent of your maximum effort Suggested speed: 3.0–3.5 mph Suggested hill grade: 0 percent
Repeat hill + rest sequence a total of 7 times	30 minutes (total)	
Cool-down	5 minutes	50–60 percent of your maximum effort Suggested speed: 2.5–3.0 mph Suggested hill grade: 0 percent
Total	**45 minutes**	

WEEK SIX: WALKING ASSIGNMENT

Goal:

In the past few weeks you've made walking a habit, experienced a faster dash, and tested yourself by marching up hills. This week we put it all together by combining all of these skills into one workout.

Mixing and matching speeds and hills is known as interval training. It's an efficient way to train because you work very hard for a period of time (which burns a lot of calories) and then rest and recover before hitting another high-intensity interval. By delaying how quickly you feel exhausted, this allows you to stretch out your workout.

This week you'll do two strolls, one speed workout, one hill workout, and one interval workout. Below is a sample "all in one shot" interval workout.

Interval	Time	Intensity
Warm-up	5 minutes	50–60 percent of your maximum effort Suggested speed: 2.5–3.0 mph Suggested hill grade: 0 percent
Interval I (speed)	10 minutes	70–80 percent of your maximum effort Suggested speed: 3.8–4.5 mph Suggested hill grade: 0–2 percent
Rest interval	5 minutes	60–70 percent of your maximum effort Suggested speed: 3.0–3.5 mph Suggested hill grade: 0 percent
Interval II (hill)	10 minutes	75–85 percent of your maximum effort Suggested speed: 3.0–3.5 mph Suggested hill grade: 4–8 percent
Rest interval	5 minutes	60–70 percent of your maximum effort Suggested speed: 3.0–3.5 mph Suggested hill grade: 0 percent
Interval III (speed)	5 minutes	75–85 percent of your maximum effort Suggested speed: 4.0–4.8 mph Suggested hill grade: 0–2 percent
Cool-down	5 minutes	50–60 percent of your maximum effort Suggested speed: 2.5–3.0 mph Suggested hill grade: 0 percent
Total	**45 minutes**	

The Perfect Beginner Body-Toning Workout

The thought of weight training scares or confuses a lot of exercise newbies. They think they will bulk up, gain weight, or injure themselves, or that they should lose some weight first before they start lifting. None of these things is true.

In fact, if you're serious about getting in shape and losing weight, then weight training must be part of your routine. Here's why.

Muscle is a very live, active tissue. That is, it requires more of your body's energy than a lethargic tissue like fat. Therefore, the more muscle you have on your body, the more calories you burn even while at rest. Studies show that for every pound of muscle, you burn an additional 30–50 calories per day. This may not sound like much, but these few extra calories are the equivalent of a three- to five-pound weight loss per year. Or, put another way, they may prevent a three- to five-pound yearly weight gain.

Though you may not lose any scale weight when you pack on a little extra muscle, you will lose inches, look smaller, and drop clothing sizes because muscle is very dense and compact. Adding muscle is the only way you can change the proportions of your body. I'm not saying you can turn yourself into a pixie if you're six feet tall or a runway model if you're naturally curvy, but having a more muscular physique can make your shoulders appear broader, your butt look tighter, and your calves more shapely in a way that nothing else—not even aerobic exercise—can.

Building muscle makes you stronger, so you can go further and faster when you do your cardio. With stronger muscles you'll go a lot longer between injuries, too.

For beginners, the term "weight training" is somewhat misleading. "Strength training" and "resistance training" are probably better terms to describe the way you will work out at first. That's because many of the exercises you do when you first start out won't require the use of much external weight. Your body weight and gravity will provide enough resistance to challenge you and increase your strength.

To start, you should do the routine below two times per week, resting at least one day in between workouts. Do one set of each of the exercises in the order they're listed. Aim for eight to fifteen repetitions per set. When the last rep is pretty easy and you're still maintaining good technique, then you can add extra weight in the form of a dumbbell or barbell. Rest as long as you need to between sets; most people find sixty to ninety seconds about right. All told, the routine will probably take you about twenty minutes to complete once you're familiar with how to do the exercises; it may take you a little longer at the beginning of your learning curve.

You should start to see changes in your body after about six weeks of regular training. Your body will look tighter, firmer, stronger. Your muscles will have more shape and definition. You may also find it easier to drop body fat. (Notice I said body *fat*, not body *weight*. Because you are building muscle at the same time you're losing fat, you may not see a difference in scale weight even though you look thinner and your clothes fit more loosely.) You'll probably feel a difference in the form of increased strength even sooner.

After six weeks of regular training, increase the number of sets to two per exercise. Keep adding weight and challenging yourself with some of the harder variations listed for each exercise whenever you're ready. You can also up your training frequency to three times per week. After about twelve weeks of regular training, you may want to cruise through some of the other chapters and consider adding some of the specialty routines to your repertoire.

■ KNEELING LEG PRESS

Muscles Worked: Buttocks and hamstrings. Your abdominals and lower back work to help you stay balanced.

Joint Cautions: Knees.

Starting Position: Get down on your elbows and knees so that your knees are directly under your hips and your elbows are directly under your shoulders. Pull your belly button in toward your spine to keep your back from sagging or arching. Tilt your chin to align your neck with the rest of your spine. Flex your left foot.

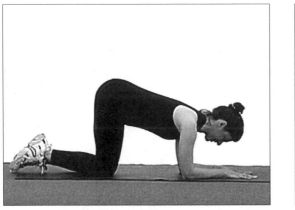 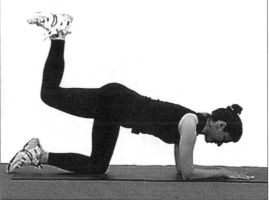

Exercise: Keeping your knee bent, lift your left leg upward until your knee is at hip height. Hold a moment as you tighten your buttocks muscles. Slowly lower to the start. Do all reps and then repeat with your right leg.

Things to Think About:

- As you press upward, imagine you are pushing a heavy object upward. You'll feel a contraction through your buttocks and back of your thigh as you press upward.
- Exhale as you push upward and inhale as you lower.
- Try to stay evenly balanced so that your body stays in a perfect square stance; don't lean all the way over to the side as you lift your leg.

Variations:

- **EASIER:** Do the exercise from a standing position, holding on to something sturdy, like the back of a large chair or a column, for support.
- **HARDER:** Place an ankle weight around your thigh or, if you have no knee problems, around your ankle. (Try one to five pounds to start.) You can also place a weight or weighted ball in the well of your knee and hold it place by squeezing your muscles as you do the exercise.
- **TO ADD INNER THIGH WORK:** As you lower, cross your thigh over the top of the other thigh and squeeze your legs together.

MODIFIED PUSH-UPS

Muscles Worked: Primarily the chest and triceps. The shoulders and abs also assist.

Joint Cautions: Shoulders, elbows, neck.

Starting Position: Get down on your hands and knees with your palms a little wider than and a little forward of your shoulders. Lift your feet and lower legs off the floor. Pull your belly button in toward your spine and tilt your chin to align your neck with the rest of your spine.

Exercise: Bend your elbows to lower yourself toward the floor. When your upper arms are parallel to the floor, push yourself upward to the starting position.

Things to Think About:
- You'll feel a strong tension through the center of your chest, the center of your shoulders, and the backs of your upper arms, especially as you straighten your arms to press upward.
- Don't allow your back to sag or your butt to stick out above the rest of your body.
- Inhale as you lower, exhale as you press upward.
- You'll feel the exercise even more if you press your hands down into the floor as you press your body upward.

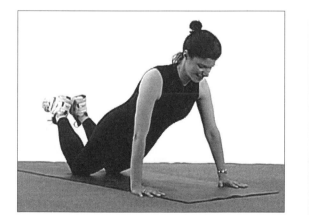 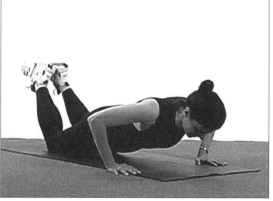

Variations:

- **EASIER:** Stand and place your palms on a wall so that they're shoulder width apart and your arms are straight. Bend your arms to lower your body toward the wall.
- **HARDER:** Straighten your legs out and balance on your toes to do a full military push-up.

PELVIC TILT

Muscles Worked: Buttocks and hamstrings. This exercise is also an excellent lower back strengthener and stretch.

Joint Cautions: None.

Starting Position: Lie on your back with your feet flat on the floor, placed about hip width apart. Pull your abs gently into your spine. Place your arms wherever comfortable.

Exercise: Gently squeeze your buttocks and tilt your hip bones forward so that your buttocks lift a few inches off the floor. Lower to the starting position, taking care not to arch your back off the floor as you do.

Things to Think About:

- To engage your hamstrings and buttocks to the max, press your feet firmly into the floor as you lift upward. You'll feel a strong pull through your buttocks, the backs of your thighs, and possibly your abdominals as you lift your buttocks off the floor.
- Exhale as you lift, inhale as you lower.
- Focus on keeping your back in contact with the floor as you move through the exercise.

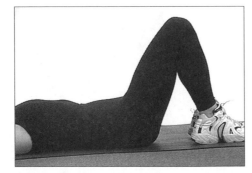 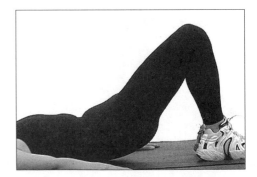

Variations:

- **TO MAKE THE EXERCISE HARDER:** Extend one leg up off the floor at a 45-degree angle as you do the pelvic tilt.
- **TO MAKE THE EXERCISE EASIER:** Place your feet a few inches farther away from your body.

■ BACK SWEEP

Muscles Worked: Upper back, shoulders, and biceps. Excellent posture awareness exercise.

Joint Cautions: Shoulder, rotator cuff.

Starting Position: Sit or stand tall while holding a light dumbbell in each hand. Pull your belly button in toward your spine to protect your lower back. Raise your arms directly over your head and cross your right wrist in front of your left.

Exercise: Gently squeeze your shoulder blades together as you lower your arms down and to the sides in an arclike path. Stop when your elbows are slightly below shoulder level, then retrace the arc back to the starting position, this time crossing your left wrist over your right

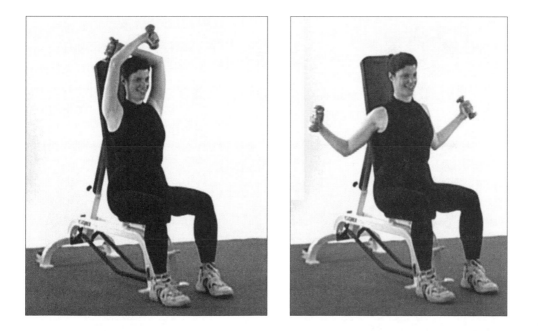

Things to Think About:
- Imagine you are wiping off a large, foggy window with your forearms. You'll feel a strong contraction through the center and tops of your shoulders as you lift and a strong contraction through the outer edges of your upper back as you lower.
- Exhale as you lower the weights, inhale as you lift.

Variations:
- EASIER: Lower the weights until they are a few inches above your shoulders, then lift back up to the start.
- HARDER: Do one arm at a time. For stability and balance, place the other hand on your hip or the seat of the chair you are sitting in.

■ HALF SQUATS

Muscles Worked: Buttocks, thighs.

Joint Cautions: Knees, lower back.

Starting Position: Stand tall with your feet a little wider than hip width apart, toes forward or angled slightly outward. Pull your belly button in toward the spine and place your hands on your hips, resting on the tops of your thighs, or held out in front of you at shoulder level—whichever you find most comfortable.

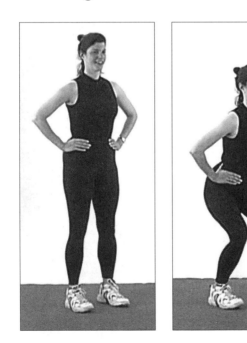

Exercise: Bend your knees four to six inches to lower your body, then carefully stand back up to the starting position.

Things to Think About:

• Imagine you are about to sit in a chair, but stand up a few inches before your butt actually touches the seat. You'll feel the front of your thigh muscles working as you stand back up; you may also feel your buttocks and the backs of your thighs working as well.

• Exhale as you lower and inhale as you stand back up.

• Don't let your knees travel forward of your toes, and avoid leaning so far forward with your upper body that you feel out of balance.

Variations:

• **EASIER:** Place a chair behind you and use it to guide your movement. You may prefer taking a stance that's wider than hip width to do this exercise. Some people feel more stable in this "plié" stance.

• **HARDER:** Bend your knees a few inches further so you lower yourself even more.

TOE RAISES

Muscles Worked: Calves.

Joint Cautions: None.

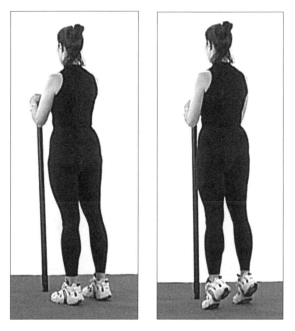

Starting Position: Stand tall with your feet hip width apart. Pull your belly button in toward your spine. Place your hands on your hips or rest them on a stable chair or some other sturdy object for support.

Exercise: Stand on your tiptoes, hold a moment, then slowly lower to the starting position.

Things to Think About:

- Pretend you are trying to peek over a tall fence. You'll feel your calf muscles contract as you stand up and stretch as you lower your heels.
- Exhale as you lift, inhale as you lower.
- Try to keep the movement fluid and straight by minimizing the amount of wobble in your ankles.

Variations:

- EASIER: Hold on to something sturdy like a wall, column, or chair for support.
- HARDER: Do the exercise with your heels hanging off the edge of a step so that, when you lower, your heels go past the starting point and you feel a stretch through your calves.

■ SHOULDER PRESS

Muscles Worked: Shoulders with some biceps and triceps involvement.

Joint Cautions: Shoulder, rotator cuff, neck.

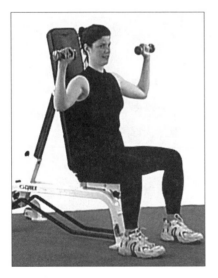

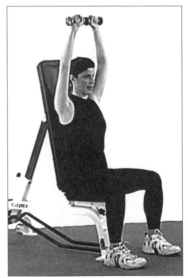

Starting Position: While holding a weight in each hand, sit up tall in a chair or workout bench (preferably one that has some back support). With your palms facing forward, bend your elbows and lift your arms up to shoulder level. Pull your belly button in toward your spine.

Exercise: Gently squeeze your shoulder blades together as you straighten your arms upward to raise the weights above your head. Lower back to the starting position.

Things to Think About:
- Your arms should travel in a steady, fixed path. You'll feel the muscles in the center and top of your shoulders contracting as you straighten your arms.
- Exhale as you lift the weights, inhale as you lower.
- Lower the weights so that your elbows are at shoulder level or slightly lower—don't go any lower than that.

Variations:
- **EASIER:** Face your palms inward. This is a good variation to do if you feel shoulder pain with other versions of the shoulder press.
- **HARDER:** Increase the weight or slow the exercise down.

■ BASIC BICEPS CURLS

Muscles Worked: Biceps.

Joint Cautions: Elbows.

Starting Position: While holding a weight in each hand, sit up tall in a chair or workout bench; if you feel you don't need back support, it's okay to sit up straight. Let your arms hang straight down at your sides with your palms facing forward. Pull your belly button in toward your spine.

Exercise: Bend your elbows to lift the weights upward toward your shoulders. Slowly lower to the starting position.

Things to Think About:
- You will feel your biceps muscles contracting as you bend your arms, especially at the midpoint of the movement.
- Don't rock backward to lift the weight.
- Exhale as you lift the weights, inhale as you lower.

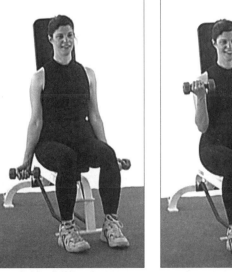
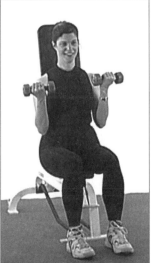

- Focus on moving slowly and with control, especially as you lower the weights.

Variations:
- **EASIER:** Do this exercise one arm at a time, alternating arms with each rep.
- **HARDER:** Do this exercise one arm at a time. Do all reps on one arm before switching to the other arm.

◼ BASIC TRICEPS DIPS

Muscles Worked: Your triceps, shoulders, and chest muscles.

Joint Cautions: Rotator cuff, shoulder, elbow, or wrist issues.

Starting Position: Sit on the edge of a stable chair with your hands on either side of you and gripping the underside of the seat. With your feet flat on the floor and hip width apart, slide your butt off the chair so that it's hovering an inch or two forward of the chair seat. Pull your belly button in toward your spine and keep your torso straight.

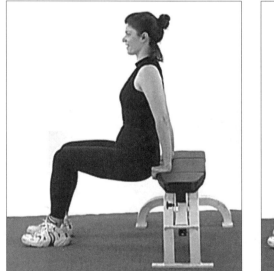
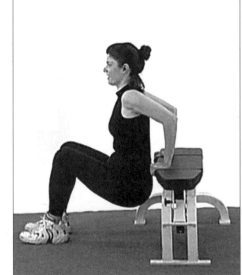

Exercise: Bend your elbows and lower your body toward the floor. When your upper arms are parallel to the floor or slightly above, press back up to the starting position.

Things to Think About:

- You'll feel this exercise very intensely in the back of your upper arms as you straighten your arms. You may feel your shoulders and the center of your chest working as well.
- Exhale as you straighten your arms and inhale as you bend.
- Make sure you are lowering yourself by bending your elbows rather than by shifting your shoulders forward and back.
- Keep your shoulders down and relaxed and don't move lower than the point at which your upper arms are parallel to the floor.

Variations:

- **EASIER:** Turn your hands sideways so they are placed fully on the bench; this is a bit easier on the wrists.
- **HARDER:** Do a Full Chair Dip as described in "The Perfect Travel Workout" on page 258.

PARTIAL AB ROLL-UP

Muscles Worked: Abdominals, lower back.

Joint Cautions: Neck, lower back.

Starting Position: Lie on your back with your knees bent, legs pressed together, and feet flat on the floor. Extend your arms over your head along the floor, palms facing in toward each other. Pull your belly button in toward your spine.

Exercise: Lift your arms off the floor, then tuck your chin to your chest. Slowly roll up and forward until your head, neck, and shoulder blades are off the floor and your arms are stretched out straight alongside your thighs. Hold a moment at the top of the movement, then slowly and carefully retrace your path back to the starting position.

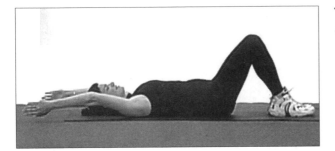

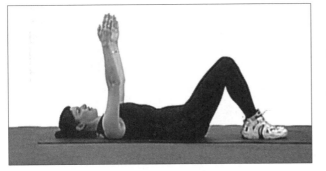

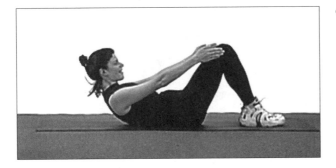

Things to Think About:

- Although this looks like a crunch or a sit-up, it is a much more focused and thorough exercise because you curl each vertebra off the floor, engaging your abdominal muscles to the max. You will feel your abs working throughout the entire exercise but especially as you reach the top of the movement.

- Exhale as you curl upward, inhale as you lower.

- Move each vertebra separately as you lift, and repaste each vertebra back in the exact same position as you lower. Avoid using momentum of any kind to initiate this movement.

- Keep your shoulders down and relaxed rather than up near your ears. Think of your arms as an extension of your upper back so that when you stretch them forward you will feel the stretch spread through your arms to the outer edge of your upper back.

Variations:

- **EASIER:** You can hold the underside of your thighs to assist yourself upward.

- **HARDER:** Curl up even higher, aiming to get your entire back off the floor and lifting yourself up to a sitting position. Again, don't use any momentum to lift!

Soreness, Cramping, and Other Aches and Pains

That dull achiness that permeates every pore. That stiffness you feel when walking downstairs. That extreme awareness of every muscle in your body. This is the so-called good pain that usually occurs a day or two after you've worked out for the first time after a long layoff or after you've pushed yourself harder than usual. Good it may be, but still—ouch.

Muscle soreness is usually characterized by a dull, generalized achiness as opposed to the sharp, very specific pain you feel when you've damaged a muscle, tendon, or ligament. There are two kinds of muscle soreness: the type you feel during or immediately after a very high-intensity workout, and the type you feel one or two days after a particularly hard workout. Immediate muscle soreness is the result of lactic acid and other by-products of muscle energy production. It usually subsides within fifteen minutes of a workout. Delayed-onset muscle soreness, or DOMS for short, is caused by microscopic tears in your muscle fibers.

While it's good to challenge yourself with exercise, if you wake up after a workout so sore that you can't comb your hair or lift your cereal spoon without assistance, you might want to rethink your workout program. If you push yourself too hard, you risk injury, overtraining, burnout, or all of the above. Here are some simple recommendations to prevent excessive soreness and how to deal with it when it does occur:

- Your body simply cannot operate at top speed after a long layoff without something breaking down. That soreness is a warning signal from your body that something has got to give. When you experience DOMS, back off for a day or two, or consider taking a few days off to let your body regroup and recoup.

- Always begin each workout with a five- or ten-minute easy warm-up to ease your body into a higher-intensity workout. This allows for a gradual elevation in body temperature and an increase in blood flow to the working muscles. To transition your body out of your workout, do five to ten minutes of easy activity as well. Good warm-ups and cool-downs include easy walking, slow jogging, light pedaling, and marching in place.

- Stretching, aspirin, and heat—all standard soreness antidotes—don't work. Try a massage instead. Although there is little scientific evidence to show that massage has any impact on muscle soreness either, many top athletes and exercise experts swear by it, and it has been proven to increase blood flow and assist the muscles in flushing out the chemical waste products that contribute to soreness on a cellular level. Whether or not it makes soreness go away faster, it feels good while you're doing it.

- Do not exercise if you experience sharp pain that's focused around a joint. This is more indicative of an injury than DOMS. If this type of pain persists for a day or two, I highly recommend a trip to a medical professional.

How Do You Judge Walking Intensity?

- At 50–60 percent of your maximum effort, your breathing should be somewhat louder and faster than at rest. You'll feel your heart beating strongly but not pounding in your chest, and you'll feel warm and slightly damp though not actually sweaty.

- At 60–70 percent of your maximum effort, your breathing will be even louder and faster. Your heart rate will speed up, too. You should be able to carry on a breathy but coherent conversation. You'll begin sweating and feeling your muscles really getting into the act.

- At 70–80 percent of your maximum effort, your breathing should sound loud and labored and you'll need to make an effort to keep it controlled and regular. You can still carry on snatches of a conversation. You will sweat liberally, your heart will be pounding in your chest, and your muscles will have to work relatively hard to sustain the effort.

- At 75–85 percent of your maximum effort, your breathing should sound loud and labored and you'll need to make an effort to keep it controlled and regular. You can barely carry on occasional snatches of a conversation. You will sweat profusely, your heart will be pounding in your chest, and your muscles will have to work very hard to sustain the effort.

Focus on Form

Review this walking technique checklist in your mind every few minutes or so. It will help you walk more efficiently and comfortably.

- **HEAD:** Keep your head up and centered between your shoulders. Keep your chin up and eyes focused straight ahead. Your head and neck should "float" above your shoulders in a relaxed, easy manner.

- **SHOULDERS:** Keep them back and down. Don't allow them to round forward or creep up toward your ears.

- **CHEST:** Your chest should feel expansive and naturally lifted.

- **ARMS:** Keep your arms low and slightly bent. Swing them easily and naturally.

- **HANDS:** Keep them loosely cupped as if you are holding a potato chip in your hand that you don't want to crush.

- **ABDOMINALS:** Pull your belly button gently in toward your spine so that you feel tall, stable, and upright. This will also protect your lower back.

- **HIPS:** Your hips should swing in a loose and natural manner. They should move forward and back rather than from side to side.

- **THIGHS:** Your walking stride should be easy and unforced, not too long and not too short. Think of your thighs as a link between your hips and your lower legs, assisting both in doing their job.

- **FEET:** Your heel will strike the ground first, then your toes will flex upward. You'll roll heel-arch-ball-toe before completing the stride and moving into the next one.

- **BREATHING AND HEART RATE:** Concentrate on keeping your breathing smooth, deep, and regular. If your breathing remains relaxed, it will help your heart beat rhythmically and steadily.

4

THE PERFECT
WEIGHT LOSS WORKOUT

To look at Nancy, you'd never know that this slip of a woman ever had a weight problem, but she did. When she went away to college, she didn't just gain the freshman fifteen—she packed twenty extra pounds onto her small frame in less than a year. Her "weight loss moment of truth" came when she was home on a break; one of her mother's friends squeezed the back of her arm and declared, "Wow, you're fat!" Nancy started with a walking program and gradually progressed to running. She lifted weights to build some muscle tone and completely overhauled her eating habits. She maintains her slim, athletic figure with an hour of exercise nearly every day plus hiking and cycling vacations whenever she and her husband, Sherman, can get away. But she still overeats from time to time. "I just exercise a little extra if I indulge," she says. "Hey, you gotta live!"

EXERCISES IN THIS CHAPTER
- Walking
- Cross Training
- Circuit Weight Training, including the following exercises:
  - Jumping Rope
  - Straddle Jumps

- Running High Steps
- Jumping Jacks
- Push-up Bridges
- Step Taps
- Punch Squats
- Lunge Pivots
- Oblique Punches
- Daffy Squats

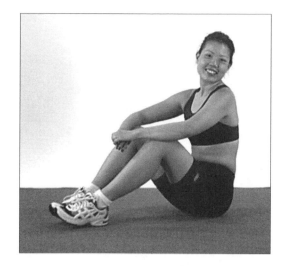

EQUIPMENT NEEDED

- Jump rope
- Step bench

ESTIMATED WORKOUT TIME

- Beginners: 30–50 minutes, five times a week
- Intermediates: 40–80 minutes, five times a week
- Advanced: 30 minutes or more, five times a week

Yogi Berra, that great American philosopher of the twentieth century, once said, "You better cut the pizza into four pieces because I'm not hungry enough to eat six." I think that about sums up how most Americans approach weight loss.

Like Berra, we haven't quite mastered the concept of portion control. We want our pizza and our extra slices too, yet continue to be absolutely amazed when the pounds pile on. We try fad diet after fad diet after fad diet with no results, and when a new fad diet hits the scene, we subscribe whole-heartedly.

We're a nation where, at any given moment, fifty-one million of us are starving ourselves with one outlandish weight loss scheme or another, yet we're getting fatter by the minute. In the 1990s, the decade that began with ultra-low-fat diets and ended with ultra-low-carb diets, the percentage of Americans considered obese nearly doubled, from 11 percent to 20 percent.

Foolish food plans aren't the only culprit. We scoop up flimsy infomercial exercise products like they're ice cream. We don't question outrageous claims like "Burn over 1,300 calories an hour!" or "Get flat, sexy abs in just three minutes a day!" We just buy, buy, buy to the tune of over $3 billion a year. And don't even get me started on the ridiculous, over-the-top claims attached to dietary supplements.

Now, I know what some of you are thinking: "But Darlene lost all that weight by doing/using/taking such and such." Yes, it's true. Some of these things do work in the short term. For instance, high-protein diets, the current darling of the diet world, may help you lose weight initially. But the majority of studies, including one sponsored by Dr. Atkins, the guru of high-protein diets himself, have found them to be ineffective when it comes to *keeping weight off in the long term*. And really, that's what we should be striving for: permanent weight loss rather than instantaneous, transitory changes.

At a Loss to Lose

I once asked a prominent weight loss researcher what weight loss method really works, once and for all. "Nothing," she replied in a fatalistic tone. I thought she was being closed-minded until I took a good look at the statistics.

Only about 5 percent of those who follow an organized weight loss plan such as Weight Watchers or Jenny Craig lose a significant amount of weight and keep it off. Some organizations, such as the Calorie Control Council, quote the percentage of successful losers as low as 1 percent.

Even such a drastic method as gastric bypass surgery, better known as stomach stapling, is successful only 50 percent of the time. Let's think about that for a minute. An invasive, risky surgical procedure that involves weeks of recovery, limits normal activity for a long period of time, and reduces the size of one's stomach to a tiny, one-ounce pouch is successful only about half of the time! (Two years after surgery an additional 10 percent of those who underwent gastric bypass and originally lost weight gain it back, so in reality the procedure has about a 40 percent success rate.)

How can we be so obsessed with shedding body fat and yet, according to every major medical source on the planet, 61 percent of us are now considered overweight, with one in five considered very overweight? What's going on here?

This is what I think is happening. Weight loss products, potions, and pills seem to have a gravitational pull all their own. We love them even though they don't work. Whether it's slick marketing, our desire for immediate success, or old-fashioned wishful thinking, we gobble up weight loss schemes even faster than we gobble up supersized portions of fried chicken. We get so sucked in by the heady promises, we readily empty our pocketbooks and put our bodies through the wringer without a second thought.

I'm laying all of this out, perhaps a little harshly, so you get the message: If you're sincere about wanting to lose weight, you need to give up the idea that there is some magical trick that will make it quick and effortless. You have to stop forking over your cash to these seductive thin-in-a-minute ploys that are designed to fatten the pocketbooks of weight loss entrepreneurs while leaving you no slimmer or healthier than you were before. Having said that, I can tell you that there is one everlasting weight loss method that is absolutely foolproof: eating less and exercising more.

Winning at Weight Loss

Michael weighed 389 pounds and knew he was at serious risk for future health problems. Though outwardly a happy guy, he was so depressed about his weight he would often come home from work and, as he puts it, "eat myself into numbness." Like most overweight people, he tried every diet known to humankind in hopes of a miracle cure. "I tried Optifast, Weight Watchers, Slim-Fast, the grapefruit diet, the mushroom diet, the cottage cheese diet, the Atkins diet, fen-phen . . . you name it," he remembers. With all that dieting, Michael's weight constantly yo-yoed; he'd lose some weight but never keep it off for very long.

When his mother told him she didn't want to lose another child (his sister had died ten years earlier), he realized it was finally time to get serious.

Michael decided to do extensive research into effective weight loss rather than impulsively embark upon yet another unproven method. Ultimately, he chose a three-month stay at Structure House, a North Carolina clinic that takes a behavioral approach to weight loss, to get himself started. While there, he received a complete reeducation about eating, lifestyle, and exercise.

"During the three months at Structure House I worked with a personal trainer once a week and did my own workouts every other day. I attended nutritional, counseling, cooking, and behavior modification classes. I also attended one-on-one personal counseling sessions. My stay resulted in losing the first seventy pounds of my hundred-and-fifty-pound weight loss," he says.

Granted, going away to a weight loss clinic is a bit extreme and probably unrealistic for many of us. But that's not the point. The point is that Michael hit upon the one proven way to lose weight safely and effectively and—here's the important part—*keep it off*. To lose weight consistently, safely, and *permanently*, you have to eat less and exercise more. You have to make a conscious effort to modify your behavior in a way that you can live with for the rest of your life—not just for a few short days, weeks, or months.

If you don't believe that simply eating less and exercising more can lead to long-term weight loss, you don't have to take my word for it. Though (believe it or not) there isn't a ton of research in this area, a few seminal studies provide backup. Consider the National Weight Control Registry, initially a three-year study that surveyed more than two thousand people who were successful at losing an average of sixty pounds and keeping it off for several years. (Our friend Michael, a participant in the study, has kept his weight off for more than five years and is still in the process of losing more.) About half the participants had been overweight since childhood, and nearly all had tried to lose weight several times before finally achieving success.

The National Weight Control Registry researchers, led by Dr. Rena Wing of the University of Pittsburgh, discovered striking similarities among the successful losers. Some of the highlights:

- Almost 100 percent of the subjects said they modified their food intake. (Note that they did not *restrict*—they *modified*.)

- About half counted calories, and about half ate the same foods they always ate but reduced portion sizes.

- Only 5 percent followed a popular diet plan (such as Atkins, the Zone, or Sugar Busters!) to lose weight. Subjects said that they failed on formal diet plans because they gave up too much responsibility for the weight loss process; most were successful when they came up with their own individual way of eating.

- Ninety-six percent of the subjects exercised regularly but did not consider themselves exercise-obsessed. (By contrast, only 22 percent of the general population reports exercising on a regular basis.)

- Subjects burned a hefty 2,800 calories a week through exercise, the equivalent of about twenty-eight miles of walking. About 80 percent burned approximately 1,000 of those calories by walking, making up the rest with cross-training activities that escalated in intensity as they continued to lose weight.

- One hundred percent of participants said that when they accepted the fact that they needed to make significant, lasting lifestyle changes in order to both lose weight and maintain that weight loss, they were successful.

There it is—the secret to lasting weight loss revealed: Eat less. Exercise more. *Forever.* I know it isn't sexy or earth-shattering or magical, but it does work. Now let's break it down in a little more detail.

The Exercise Paradox

Exercise seems to be the number one predictor of who will succeed and who will fail at the weight loss game. Those who exercise succeed. Those who don't fail. It's not just the conclusion of the National Weight Control Registry, either. Scores of studies have yielded similar findings. For example, a recent survey of thirty-two thousand *Consumer Reports* readers, though not a study per se, found that eight out of ten weight loss winners listed exercise as their number one strategy, with an eyebrow-raising 29 percent adding weight lifting to their repertoire.

That exercise is a big key to weight loss is actually somewhat surprising because, when you come right down to it, exercise doesn't burn that many calories.

Take running, for example. At a calorie burn of roughly 8–14 calories per minute (depending on your body weight and how fast you run), it's a pretty intense activity. If you run for thirty minutes, a respectable workout for most of us, you might burn about 300 calories. Now, consider how easy it is to chow down the same number of calories. That glass of orange juice and two slices of buttered toast you had for breakfast (375 calories) will get you there and then some. Even if you run the traditional marathon distance of 26.2 miles, you'd only burn about 2,600 calories. With Big Macs, doughnuts, and french fries the mainstay of the average American diet, most of us easily scarf down that number of calories on an average day.

So why is exercise such an integral part of the long-term weight loss process? The truth is, we're not quite sure. However, we can speculate.

Even though the number of calories you incinerate from working up a good sweat may not be very high in comparison to how easily you can take them in, every little bit seems to help. It appears that even small variations in calorie balance can have a big impact on weight. Just a 50-calorie difference per day either way can theoretically result in a yearly weight fluctuation of three to five pounds.

Exercise also causes your metabolism to elevate slightly because it results in increased muscle mass and decreased body fat (weight training appears to have the biggest effect on your muscle-to-fat ratio). Muscle is a much more active tissue than fat; one pound of muscle burns approximately 20 percent more calories than one pound of fat. While this may result in a metabolic increase of only about 30 calories per pound of extra muscle per day, again, every little bit helps.

Some experts speculate that regular exercisers are simply more health-conscious overall. Exercise seems to correlate with other healthy lifestyle habits, such as mindful eating, limited alcohol intake, and not smoking. Good health habits are positively associated with lower body weight.

But perhaps the biggest paradox regarding exercise is that activities that burn the most calories aren't necessarily the best ones for weight loss. Walking burns only about 5 calories per minute, yet more than 80 percent of National Weight Control Registry participants walked as their primary means of exercise. It could be that because walking is easy to do for long periods of time and rarely results in any injuries, you can simply keep at it longer without any interruptions.

All this is an educated guess. We don't have a definitive answer on why exercise is so important for losing weight and maintaining weight loss, but we are sure that it works. The workout routine I will give you a little later in this chapter is patterned after tried-and-true weight loss workout plans.

Losing Propositions

Obviously, as the National Weight Control Registry and other studies have demonstrated, healthy eating plays an integral part in the weight loss process. But what does healthy eating mean? Clearly it means different things to different people, including different nutritional experts.

Some people believe that you need to eat high-protein meals for weight loss, while others insist that low-fat is the way to go. Some say to chew on raw meat and earthy roots the way cave dwellers did, while others say to follow the same diet as their favorite movie star. There are theories on everything—from snacking more to snacking less, from starving yourself to stuffing yourself. Some say to eat certain foods to speed up weight loss, while others say to avoid those very same foods.

Confusing? It can be. But it doesn't have to be. While I'm not a registered dietician, I do consider myself a highly educated consumer. So while we wait for the nutrition authorities to sort it all out, let me tell you what I think.

What to eat involves some pretty simple concepts when you get right down to it. Through experience and speaking to other experts, I've distilled the concept of healthy eating for weight loss down to six basic truths. I think you need to take these rules and use them to customize your diet in a way that works for you. If you do so, I promise you that you won't have to rearrange your entire life to revolve around food.

- **Portion control.** It's not necessary to pile your plate up to the ceiling or have food spill over the sides. Eat everything in moderation. Don't feel obligated to clean your plate. A portion is equivalent to something the size of your fist, not the size of your head. For accurate portion sizes, read labels; if you must, get out a food scale and measure things for a while until you can eyeball accurately. You may be surprised to find what a true portion size really looks like. Take spaghetti. The typical portion you're served in a restaurant is often three to four times the suggested serving size listed on the back of the Ronzoni box. I think this may be how carbohydrates got a bad name all of a sudden. There isn't any scientific proof that they're more fattening in moderation than other foods—we're just eating too much of them.

- **Eat five fruits and veggies a day.** Fruits and vegetables are high in vitamins and nutrition yet low in calories. They're packed with fiber to help you feel full and satisfied. Aim to eat a variety of foods in these two groups every day. Numerous studies show that eating ample amounts of fruit and vegetables helps you lose weight by helping you feel full on fewer calories.

- **Avoid processed, junk, and fast foods.** Limit foods with high sugar and white flour content. Steer clear of foods that are packed with unpronounceable ingredients. Try to eat foods as close to their natural state as possible. Some examples: an apple is a better choice than apple juice; boiled new potatoes are a better choice than french fries; raw carrots are a better choice than carrot cake.

- **Forget shortcuts.** Oh, I know I've told you this about a thousand times already, but it bears repeating: no fad diets! I don't care which of your friends lost twenty pounds in three days or which star overhauled her body on what diet. Fad diets wreak havoc on your metabolism and leave you feeling discouraged. They may work in the short term but they are never, *never* a long-term solution.

- **Forgive your mistakes and get on with it.** We all have bad days. It's what you do the next day—and the days to follow—that will make or break your efforts. If you binge or overeat one day (or even one meal), forgive yourself and get back on the wagon. Don't let one mistake spiral into long-term failure.

- **It's all about the calories.** Forget all of the pseudoscientific theories that say otherwise. The sooner you accept this fact and begin adjusting your diet and exercise accordingly, the sooner you will see success.

Your Perfect Weight Loss Exercise Plan

THREE-PHASE EXERCISE PLAN

The plan that follows is based on what research has shown to be successful. I've divided it into three five-week phases with the assumption that you're starting from scratch and need a gradual buildup into the full routine. If you're further along than that, you can skip to the second or third phase right away. The caloric counts I give you are based on a 150-pound person. If you're lighter, you'll burn fewer calories, and if you're heavier, you'll burn more.

Phase One, the first five weeks, starts out with a basic walking program to build up your base of stamina and begin the weight loss process. You'll then kick up the intensity in Phase Two by adding circuit training and increased walking duration into the mix (I'll describe how to do the circuit training in the next section). In Phase Three you'll cut back on the number of days you walk, continue to circuit-train several days a week, and add in some higher-intensity cross-training days. Once you reach the end of Phase Three you can continue with the same program or add some of the other programs in this book.

This plan takes commitment and patience. If you follow my tips on eating for weight loss and use the tips in the "A Few Small Steps in the Right Direction" sidebar on page 89, you should experience a one-to-three-pound weekly weight loss. That's a lot slower than you may be used to if you've been a fad diet addict up until now, but if you lose weight any quicker, you wind up losing more water and precious muscle mass than fat.

PHASE ONE

Strategy:

Brisk walking five days a week for five weeks. Each week, increase walking time by five minutes per session so that you are burning a total of 120 additional calories weekly.

Week I	Total walking time	Intensity
Day I	30 minutes	Moderate pace
Day 2	30 minutes	Moderate pace
Day 3	Rest	
Day 4	30 minutes	Moderate pace
Day 5	30 minutes	Moderate pace
Day 6	30 minutes	Moderate pace
Day 7	Rest	
Total calorie burn for the week =		**750 calories**

Continue to walk five days/week	Increase in walking time	Total walking time	Calories burned for the week
Week 2	5 minutes	35 minutes	840 calories
Week 3	5 minutes	40 minutes	960 calories
Week 4	5 minutes	45 minutes	1,080 calories
Week 5	5 minutes	50 minutes	1,200 calories

PHASE TWO: GET IN GEAR

Strategy:

Exercise five days a week for the next five weeks. Increase overall exercise time from Phase One; introduce the circuit-training routine described in this chapter. Increase your total calorie burn by approximately 100–200 calories a week.

Week 6	Exercise plan	Intensity
Day 1	Walk: 40 minutes Circuit training: 20 minutes	Moderate pace High intensity
Day 2	Walk: 40 minutes	Moderate pace
Day 3	Rest	
Day 4	Walk: 40 minutes Circuit training: 20 minutes	Moderate pace High intensity
Day 5	Walk: 40 minutes	Moderate pace
Day 6	Walk: 40 minutes	High/moderate-intensity interval workout
Day 7	Rest	
Total calorie burn for the week =		**1,300 calories**

Continue to exercise five days/week	Increase in length of workout	Total activity time	Calories burned for the week
Week 7	Duration of each walk: 3 minutes Circuit training: 10 minutes	43 minutes 30 minutes	1,500
Week 8	Duration of each walk: 4 minutes Circuit training: no increase	47 minutes 30 minutes	1,600
Week 9	Duration of each walk: 3 minutes Circuit training: no increase	50 minutes 30 minutes	1,700
Week 10	Duration of each walk: 5 minutes Circuit training: no increase	55 minutes 30 minutes	1,800

PHASE THREE: PUMP IT UP

Strategy:

Exercise five days a week for five weeks. Walk three times a week at a moderate pace; continue to circuit-train; introduce higher-intensity cross-training activities into your routine. The amount of time you spend exercising depends on the cross-training activity you choose to do. Use the "Cross-Training Calorie Burn" chart on page 77 to determine how many calories the fitness activity of your choice burns.

Week 11	Exercise	Intensity
Day 1	Walk: 30 minutes	Moderate pace
	Circuit training: 30 minutes	High intensity
Day 2	Cross-training activity	Burn 500 calories
Day 3	Rest	
Day 4	Walk: 30 minutes	Moderate pace
	Circuit training: 30 minutes	High Intensity
Day 5	Cross-training activity	Burn 500 calories
Day 6	Walk: 30 minutes	Moderate pace
	Cross-training activity	Burn 500 calories
Day 7	Rest	
Total calorie burn for the week =		**2,100 calories**

Continue to exercise five days/week	Increase in length of workout	Total activity time	Calories burned for the week
Week 12	Duration of each walk: 5 minutes	35 minutes	2,300 calories
	Calorie burn of each cross-training session: no increase		500 calories

Continue to exercise five days/week	Increase in length of workout	Total activity time	Calories burned for the week
Week 13	Duration of each walk: 5 minutes Calorie burn of each cross-training session: no increase	40 minutes	2,500 calories 500 calories
Week 14	Duration of each walk: 5 minutes Calorie burn of each cross-training session: 50 calories	40 minutes	2,600 calories 550 calories
Week 15	Duration of each walk: 5 minutes Calorie burn of each cross-training session: no increase	45 minutes	2,800 calories 550 calories

CROSS-TRAINING CALORIE BURN

Activity	To burn 500 calories	To burn 550 calories
	35 minutes	40 minutes
Run		
Play squash		
Jump rope		
	45 minutes	50 minutes
Aerobics class (high intensity)		
Kickboxing		
Martial arts		
Swim laps		
Cross-country ski machine		
Cycling (fast)		
	50 minutes	57 minutes
Jog		
Race walking		
Circuit weight training		
Tennis (singles)		

Activity	To burn 500 calories	To burn 550 calories
	60 minutes	**65 minutes**
Aerobics class (moderate intensity)		
Cycling (moderate)		
Skating and blading		
Step aerobics		
	70 minutes	**78 minutes**
Dancing		
Hiking		
Rowing		
Stair climber (moderate)		
Water aerobics		
Golf (carrying clubs)		
Tennis (doubles)		

Circuit Training

Circuit training consists of doing a series of exercises one after the other with little or no rest in between sets. This type of high-speed routine is a sort of cardio-strength hybrid with a couple of advantages: You burn a ton of calories in a short period of time, and though you don't get quite the cardio or toning results you would if you separated the two, you still develop a decent amount of both stamina and strength.

When you first begin doing the circuit-training routine outlined in this chapter (week six), you'll do approximately two sets of each exercise. Rather than counting reps, go for time, one minute each set. Move from exercise to exercise with no break in between if you can, but if you can't, try to keep the time between sets to under thirty seconds. Rather than doing two sets of the same exercise in a row, do the entire routine once through, then swing around to the beginning and repeat the sequence.

Starting at week seven, you'll up the circuit time to approximately thirty minutes or three sets per exercise. (If you're not ready to up your circuit-training intensity, don't worry about it. Stick with the twenty-minute routine until you can do it comfortably and then bump it up.) Again, you'll do each move for a minute and take little or no rest in between. Complete the entire sequence, then take it from the top. For each strength-training exercise, use a weight (when needed) that feels challenging but still allows you to complete the full minute comfortably.

THE PERFECT WEIGHT LOSS CIRCUIT ROUTINE

JUMPING ROPE

Muscles Worked: This is an intense full-body workout.

Joint Cautions: Knees, shoulders, ankles.

Starting Position: Hold an end of the rope in each hand and stand tall with your feet together in front of the rope line. Bend your elbows and hold your arms out to the sides at about hip level.

Exercise: Spin the rope at a fairly quick speed and, as it approaches your toes, skip over it. Keep your heels lifted and jump off the balls of your feet. Stay low—only jump an inch or so off the floor—and when you land, allow knees to bend slightly to help absorb the impact.

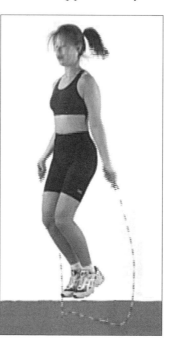

Things to Think About:
- Most people feel this exercise in every muscle of their body but especially the shoulders, wrists, and calves.
- Avoid double-hopping over the rope; one jump per turn will feel smoother and more natural. Spinning the rope at least seventy turns per minute will help you get into the rhythm.
- Land as softly as possible, making sure to keep a slight give in your knees as you jump.

Variations:

- **EASIER:** Hold the rope in one hand and spin it at your side as you jump in rhythm.
- **HARDER:** Spin rope and, as it approaches your toes, shift your weight slightly to the left, move left foot a small distance forward, and jump, again staying low and slightly bending knees on touchdown. On the next spin, shift your weight right. Continue alternating.

■ STRADDLE JUMPS

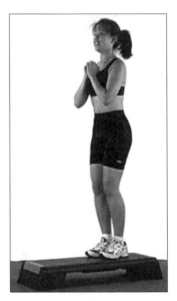

Muscles Worked: A great lower-body exercise that especially targets the calves, the front and back of the thighs, the inner and outer thighs, and the buttocks.

Joint Cautions: Slight knee caution.

Starting Position: Place up to two sets of risers underneath your step. Stand tall on top of the platform facing toward one end with your feet together and your arms bent to 90 degrees at your sides.

Exercise: Bend your knees a few inches. Spring up a small way, and as you do, spread your legs apart so that you land softly on the floor with your feet on either side of the platform. Bend your knees a few inches again and spring back up to the starting position on top of the platform. Keep your arms stationary or use them to help power the movement, whichever feels more comfortable.

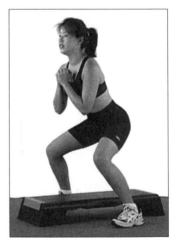

Things to Think About:

- Imagine the step and floor are very hot and you need to jump up to avoid burning your feet. You'll feel most of the work being done by the front of your thighs and your calves as you land from your jumps.

Variations:

- **EASIER:** Step down with your right foot to the side of the step, then your left foot to the other side. Return your right foot to the top of the step, then your left.
- **HARDER:** As you jump off the platform, bend your knees into a full squat before jumping back up to the starting position.

■ RUNNING HIGH STEPS

Muscles Worked: Your calves, thighs, and buttocks get a great workout here.

Joint Cautions: Mild knee caution.

Starting Position: Stand tall with your feet together and your elbows bent, arms held at your sides at waist level.

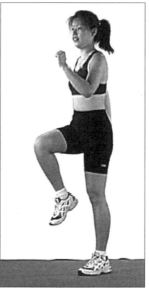

Exercise: Staying up on the balls of your feet, run in place, bringing your knees up high and using a vigorous arm swing.

Things to Think About:

- You'll feel your calves plus the fronts and backs of your thighs working the entire time.
- Land softly, taking care to land evenly across the balls of your feet.

Variations:

- **EASIER:** Instead of running in place, march in place.
- **HARDER:** Instead of running in place, *sprint* in place.

▓ JUMPING JACKS

Muscles Worked: This is a high-energy exercise that works every muscle in your body.

Joint Cautions: Knees, hips.

Starting Position: Stand tall with your feet together and your arms down at your sides.

Exercise: Keeping your knees springy and pressing off the balls of your feet, jump up a small distance and land so that your legs move apart a comfortable distance as your arms reach up and over your head. Immediately jump back to the start. Reps should be continuous.

Things to Think About:
- This is a high-intensity exercise you'll feel just about everywhere in your body!
- How far you move your legs apart depends on your comfort level. Most people will land with their feet slightly wider than hip width apart.
- It's important to stay on the balls of your feet and keep your knees springy to protect your joints.

Variations:
- **EASIER:** Do a half jack, only lifting your arms up to just below shoulder level.
- **HARDER:** As you jump back to the start, cross one ankle in front of the other and cross one wrist in front of the other.

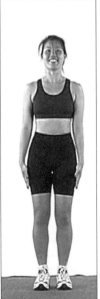
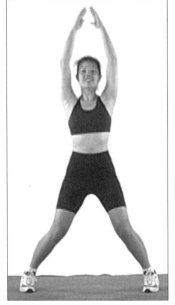

■ PUSH-UP BRIDGES

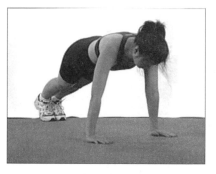

Muscles Worked: An intense move that targets your chest, shoulders, triceps, and abdominals.

Joint Cautions: Shoulders, rotator cuff, elbows, lower back.

Starting Position: Lie on your stomach with your legs out straight, feet a few inches apart. Bend your elbows and place your palms on the floor slightly to the side and in front of your shoulders. Straighten your arms and press your body upward so that your arms are nearly straight and you're balanced on your palms and the underside of your toes. Tuck your chin a few inches toward your chest so that your forehead faces the floor. Pull your abdominal muscles inward.

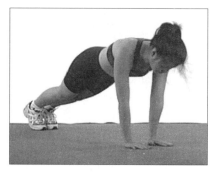

Exercise: Lift your left hand up and place it down next to your right hand. Next, move your left foot next to your right foot. Then lift your right hand up and move it out so that your hands are once again shoulder width apart. Finally, move your right foot out to the side so your legs are once again apart. After "walking" three "steps" in one direction, "walk" three "steps" back to your starting point.

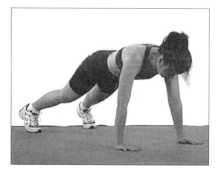

Things to Think About:
- You will feel this exercise through the entire range of motion, mainly in the outer edges of your chest, your shoulders, and the backs of your arms. Your abs will contract more strongly toward the end of the set.
- It's important to keep your shoulders relaxed and your elbows slightly bent to avoid undo stress on your joints.

Variations:
- **EASIER:** Balance on your knees to do the move.
- **HARDER:** Do a push-up between reps. Pop a few inches off the floor and land; alternate landing with your hands together, then apart.

■ STEP TAPS

Muscles Worked: This high-intensity exercise works your thighs and calves. Because you swing your arms, it also works your shoulders.

Joint Cautions: Mild knee caution.

Starting Position: Place up to two sets of risers underneath your step platform. Stand tall in front of the center of your step with your feet together and your arms bent to 90 degrees.

Exercise: In a running cadence, lean back very slightly and tap the toe of your left foot on the edge of a step. Lower it back down as you lift your right toe up to tap the edge of the step. Swing your arms in opposition to help keep your balance and to help keep the movement fluid. Taps should be rhythmic and continuous.

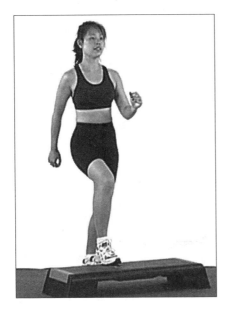

Things to Think About:
- The rhythm of this exercise is a quick running in place. You'll feel the muscles in the front and back of your thighs plus your calves contracting the entire time. The tension in your muscles will build throughout the duration of the set.

Variations:
- **EASIER:** Rather than doing this at a running pace, do it at a marching pace.
- **HARDER:** Tap your heel on the step rather than your toe. Use a lower step for this version.

■ PUNCH SQUATS

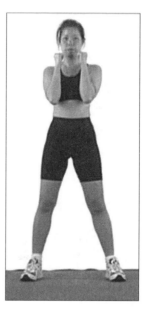

Muscles Worked: A total-body exercise.

Joint Cautions: Knees.

Starting Position: Stand tall with your feet a few inches wider than hip width apart, your toes turned out slightly, and your abdominals contracted. With your arms bent, make fists and raise your hands to your ears with your palms facing inward. Bend your knees slightly.

Exercise: Alternate left and right punches across your body at chest level as you gradually lower into a squat position. Rotate your palm downward as you punch out and rotate it back to an inward position as you pull your arm back in. Stand back up and repeat.

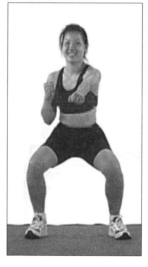

Things to Think About:
- Pretend you're a boxer trying to punch while you duck to avoid being hit. You'll feel all of your muscles working, but especially your shoulders as you punch outward and your thighs as you stand back up.
- Avoid allowing your knees to travel in front of your toes.
- Punch by twisting from the waist and powering from the shoulder; avoid snapping your elbows.

Variations:
- **EASIER:** Do the punches and skip the squats.
- **HARDER:** Increase the speed of your punching as you squat and add punches as you stand back up.

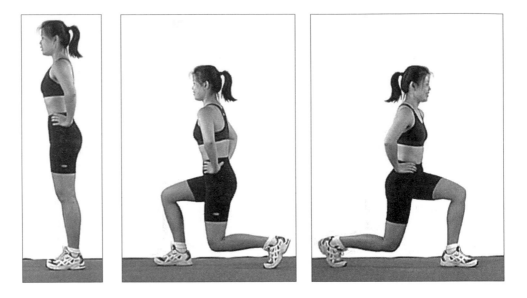

■ LUNGE PIVOTS

Muscles Worked: This exercise is powered by all of your lower-body muscles as well as your abdominals. You'll also challenge your sense of balance and coordination.

Joint Cautions: Knee, lower back.

Starting Position: Stand tall with your feet hip width apart and your hands on your hips. Pull your abdominals inward.

Exercise: Step your right foot about a stride's length forward and bend both knees until your right thigh is parallel to the floor and your left thigh is perpendicular to it. As soon as you lower into the lunge, twist from the balls of your feet so that you are facing in the other direction and both legs straighten out several inches; your left foot will now be in front. From this position stand back up and begin the next repetition with your left leg.

Things to Think About:
• The pivot is quick, like someone surprised you from behind and you're turning around to see who it is. You'll feel this exercise in your but-

tocks and thighs as you lower, and in the outer part of your hips as you pivot. You'll also feel a strong contraction in the front of your thighs as you stand back up.

- Look up so you don't tip forward; keep your abs strong, especially as you pivot.
- Don't allow your knees to extend past your toes.

Variations:
- **EASIER:** Do lunges as described on page 255.
- **HARDER:** Add some arm movement to this exercise. As you pivot, punch out with one arm and bring the other one in toward your chin.

■ OBLIQUE PUNCHES

Muscles Worked: This is an incredibly focused move for all your abdominal and lower back muscles. It also works your upper-body muscles.

Joint Cautions: Mild lower back caution.

Starting Position: Stand tall with your feet a few inches wider than hip width apart. Bend your arms to 90 degrees and hold them at your sides at waist level. Make fists with both hands with your palms facing upward. Bend your knees slightly and pull your abs strongly inward to brace the center of your body.

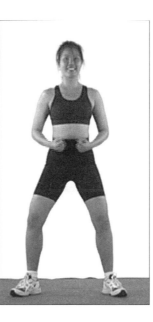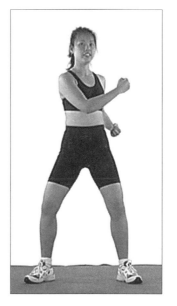

Exercise: Maintaining that braced middle and bent elbows, twist from the middle and punch your right arm across your body to the left at waist level. Move through the starting position and punch your left arm to the right. Continue alternating punches.

Things to Think About:
- Imagine your middle is like a wet towel and you are wringing out all the water. You will feel your abdominals working the entire time.
- The key to this exercise is keeping your abs pulled in strongly and the rest of your body stable.

Variations:
- **EASIER:** Rather than punching, reach across your body with straighter arms and open hands.
- **HARDER:** Hold light dumbbells as you punch.

■ DAFFY SQUATS

Muscles Worked: This is an awesome buttocks, hip, and thigh workout that also challenges your sense of balance and coordination.

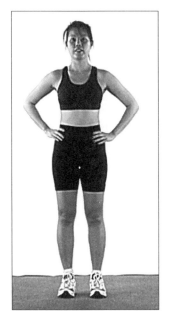

Joint Cautions: Knees, lower back.

Starting Position: Stand tall with your feet hip width apart, your hands on your hips, and your abdominals contracted.

Exercise: Step your right foot back behind you at an angle until your right knee is diagonally in line with your left heel.

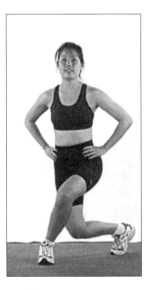

Bend your knees until your left thigh is parallel to the floor and your right thigh bends a comfortable distance. Stand back up to the starting position and repeat to the left. Continue alternating left and right reps.

Things to Think About:
- This exercise resembles an exaggerated curtsey. You'll feel your thighs working as you stand back up to the start. You may also feel a contraction in your inner and outer thighs.

- Move slowly and carefully to maintain your balance.
- Be very careful to keep your knees directly above your toes; don't allow your knees to press inward or outward.

Variations:

- **EASIER:** Stick with a squats exercise as described on page 254.
- **HARDER:** Use your arms to help power the movement. Raise them out to the sides as you lunge.

A Few Small Steps in the Right Direction

Did you know that doodling, twisting paper clips, and tapping your toes can help you lose weight? Studies show that world-class fidgeters can burn up to 800 extra calories per day. This is in line with the surgeon general's recommendations on getting thirty minutes of accumulated activity daily for better health and to aid in the weight loss process. Those same studies also show that about 40 percent of those who achieve weight loss success increase the simple physical activities in their daily routines.

A few calories here and a few calories there can make a significant dent in your weight. Some simple ways to increase your daily activity:

- Fidgeting for five minutes by tapping your toes and doodling while you're on the phone: 15 calories

- Window shopping for ten minutes: 35 calories

- A quick run through your garden to pull some weeds: 60 calories

- Lugging your toddler around the house for five to six minutes: 40 calories

- Forgoing an escalator and walking up one flight of stairs: 16 calories/flight

- Vacuuming for ten minutes: 40 calories

- Singing "We Are the World" at a karaoke bar: 20.7 calories

My Mother's Thighs

Do you look like your mother right down to those saddlebags at the top and sides of your thighs? Feel free to blame her for your weight loss woes, but only partially. While you do share genes with your mother, as well as all of your other relatives, about 40 percent of how far you tip the needle on the bathroom scale is due to environmental factors such as eating, exercise, and lifestyle. And scientists aren't sure how much of the genetic component attributed to weight loss (and gain) may be the result of shared health habits among family members.

Studies done on adopted children and identical twins reared in different homes do show that body weight can be strongly influenced by genetics. However, most experts agree that using your family history of "fat genes" as an excuse for being overweight is a cop-out. By changing your eating habits, exercising, and making other positive behavioral changes, you can and will lose weight. You may have to try a little harder if being big runs in the family, but it's not impossible to overcome your size inheritance.

Sizing Yourself Up

Your body weight is only part of the picture. Body fat percentage is probably a better indicator of whether or not you should drop a few pounds because it gives you an idea of how much of your weight is fat and how much is muscle. According to the American College of Sports Medicine, 16–26 percent body fat is optimal for a woman; for a man, the optimal figure is 12–20 percent. (Women carry more essential fat for childbearing purposes.)

The most common way to measure body fat is with fat calipers, a device that looks like a freakishly large pair of salad tongs. An experienced tester, usually a trainer, doctor, or nurse, pinches you with the calipers on several different places on your body and then plugs the sum of your skin fold measurements into a formula to determine your body fat. This method is full of inaccuracies and is probably only as good as the person doing the pinching, but it's useful for comparative purposes as you go through your weight loss process. It's a good idea to retest your body fat percentage every three months or so.

Other ways to measure body fat include underwater weighing, where you are dunked in a large vat of water to see how dense your body is (the more fat, the less dense), and running low level currents of electricity through your body, again to measure density.

Beyond body fat, there are several other methods for assessing the healthiness of your current weight, including body mass index, which takes into account your weight as it relates to your height, and waist-to-hip ratio. It doesn't really matter which weight assessment method you subscribe to so long as you monitor yourself consistently.

5

THE PERFECT ABDOMINAL WORKOUT

Heather grew up on a farm in Minnesota where chores such as chopping and stacking wood were a part of everyday life. That plus a dad who encouraged her to do push-ups and sit-ups helped shape her small yet curvy figure. She has abs to die for but admits she has to work at it. "If I don't do abdominal exercises, yoga, and Pilates, my abs tend to be weak," she confesses. Heather thinks having a strong, fit middle can change your appearance in more ways than one. "Sure, a flat stomach looks great, but more important, good ab muscles improve your posture. When you sit and stand up straighter it gives you an elongated look," she says. Heather also thinks that if you want a sculpted middle, simply doing abdominal exercises won't cut it. "You also have to eat right and do regular cardio workouts to burn calories," she advises.

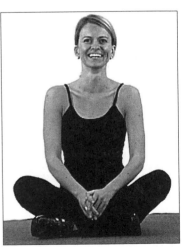

EXERCISES IN THIS CHAPTER

- Standing Ab Awareness
- Ball Roll-ups
- Posture Lifts
- Ab Pendulums
- Slow Bicycles

- Ab Lifts
- Mini Leg Lowers
- Hundreds
- Hover
- Ball Curls

EQUIPMENT NEEDED

- Physioball

ESTIMATED WORKOUT TIME

- Beginners: 5–10 minutes, two or three times a week
- Intermediates: 10–15 minutes, two or three times a week
- Advanced: 15–20 minutes, two or three times a week

A gentle breeze blows a piece of paper to the floor. You stretch forward to pick it up. You miss it and spend the next several seconds twisting and adjusting your body as the breeze blows the paper in a spiral path around you. Finally you arch backward and catch it just before it floats over your head.

Stretch, twist, arch, curl. Your middle muscles, as I like to call the muscles that wrap around your torso, are the muscles responsible for all of the spinal motion it took for you to retrieve that errant paper. This three-dimensional action is the way you typically use your abdominal muscles in real life.

For instance, the rectus abdominis—the long, flat sheet of muscle that runs the length of your torso—powers all forward-bending, crunch-style movements; the internal and external obliques, which wrap around your waist, initiate twists and bends to the side; the erector spinae, the muscles of your lower back, arch the spine backward; and the transversus abdominis, which resides underneath the rectus abdominis, is used for powerful exhalation. Together, these middle muscles work as a team to support your spine as you move your torso (such as when your muscles pull inward and stretch as you twist around in your seat to reach for something behind you) or when your middle needs to remain strong and still as you move some other part of your body (such as protecting your lower back and preventing extraneous movement when you throw a ball).

Stabilization and support are the main jobs of the middle muscles in everyday life. That's why I believe it's important to train your middle muscles to do these jobs well.

The abdominal workout you've been doing at the gym or that's featured in your favorite exercise video is probably far too one-dimensional, in my opinion. The traditional ab workout usually concentrates on the isolated actions of each muscle rather than the concepts of muscle teamwork, stabilization, and support.

Variations on the abdominal crunch exercise are typically the foundation of most ab training programs. While there is nothing wrong with lying on your back and curling the top half of your body off the floor, it's certainly not the most effective way to train your middle, and it won't even necessarily do a good job of strengthening, flattening, or toning once you build a certain amount of basic strength.

This opinion is backed up by science. Recently, researchers at the Biomechanics Lab at San Diego State University tested more than a dozen popular ab moves and gadgets to see how they stacked up in terms of muscle usage, safety, and efficiency. The result? Crunches finished somewhere near the bottom of useful ab exercises. And if you think about it, it makes sense. How many situations in life call for you to bend forward twenty times in quick succession?

The San Diego State University researchers found that the best abdominal exercises are the ones that ask your muscles to act in concert with one another to keep the spine stable, still, and in alignment. The exercises in this chapter either scored somewhere near the top of the list or are inspired by the same effective principles.

Abdominal-Training Misconceptions

Before we leave the idea of doing crunches as your primary ab workout behind and get into my no-crunch ab-training program, I'd like to take a little time to dispel some common myths about abdominal training by answering several commonly asked questions. People seem to be more confused about the rights and wrongs of ab training than they are about programming their VCRs.

HOW DO I WORK MY LOWER ABS?

There has long been a misconception that there are "upper" and "lower" abs, but as I told you in the introduction to this chapter, your rectus abdominis is one long, flat sheet of muscle that runs from the bottom of the breastbone to the top of the pelvis. You work the whole muscle with virtually any abdominal exercise you do. If you want to kick in more of those lower fibers, concentrate on keeping your abs pulled in tight as you do each repetition regardless of what exercise you're working on; focus especially on keeping that "cummerbund" region below the belly button pulled inward. Some people seem to grasp this concept right away, while others need some practice to build up enough control and awareness to maximize the work effort of these lower fibers. I talk more about this concept in the how-to section of this chapter and within each exercise description.

IS DOING A LOT OF TRAINING EVERY DAY THE ONLY WAY TO GET FLAT ABS?

For some reason many people think that they have to spend hours and hours working their abs to get results. "Not so," says Grace De Simone, a certified personal trainer who is well known in the fitness industry for teaching other trainers how to train. "More is not better. Quality is more important than quantity. You should work each repetition as if it's the only one you are going to do." Good advice.

I don't know how the high-repetition myth got started, but I can tell you this: Doing a thousand repetitions every day will not give you better results, though it will probably cause backaches and abdominal strains. Like any other muscle, work your abs two to four times a week, giving them at least a day's rest in between workouts. Do three to ten sets per workout, eight to fifteen repetitions per set. As De Simone says, make each rep count, so that by the end of each set you feel like you gave it your all.

WHICH EXERCISE IS BEST FOR
PEELING THE FAT OFF MY MIDDLE?

Your abs respond to training just like any other muscle; work them properly and consistently and you'll be rewarded with a middle that's firmer and tighter. However, don't expect to melt away tummy fat by doing ab exercises. You simply can't spot-reduce this or any other area of your body. The only way to reduce middle-body fat is by combining a sensible diet with aerobic exercise—and even then there's no guarantee you'll lose the weight where you want to lose it.

HOW DO I GET WASHBOARD ABS?

The appearance of your middle muscles has a lot to do with heredity, skin tone, whether or not you tend to store fat around your middle, life experiences, and a whole list of other factors too numerous to mention. You can do everything right but still not have the flat, sculpted six-pack of your dreams. Does that mean you shouldn't exercise your abs? Of course not! Working your abs makes them stronger, thereby flatter and tighter-looking; stronger abs also add up to better posture and a reduced risk of chronic back pain. Just have realistic expectations about what look you can and can't achieve.

WHICH AB GADGET WORKS BEST?

The myth that you need some gizmo or device to properly train your abdominals has made millionaires out of Suzanne Somers and other informercial hucksters. The answer is that none of them works best because the best exercises you can do for your abs require no special equipment. The San Diego State University study ranked several popular ab gadgets, including the Ab Roller and Torso Track, near the bottom of the effectiveness list. The only ab exercise done with a prop that was highly ranked was the Ball Curl, which is done on an oversized ball called a physioball. I've included that exercise in this chapter.

Proper Ab-Training Principles

Simply slapping through a series of ab exercises—even the right ab exercises—will not be very effective. How you do your ab moves is just as important as the moves you do. Impeccable technique is crucial. As you do the exercises in this chapter, I want you to keep the following technique pointers in mind at all times.

First of all, slow things down. Take the time to truly feel your muscles working. If you can do more than the highest number of repetitions suggested per set, then either you're not doing them correctly or the exercise is too easy. Strive for good technique and experiment until you find a combination of exercises that offers a properly intense workout.

Proper breathing is another key to successful abdominal training. By exhaling strongly through your mouth as you exert an effort and inhaling through your nose as you release an effort, you work deep muscle fibers of the transverse abdominals that would not otherwise get into the act. Note that some of the exercises in this chapter are stationary, so the trick is to breathe deeply in and out as you hold the position.

How much rest should you take between sets? As little as you can stand. Ideally, you should be able to flow from one exercise to another without taking any break at all. Don't worry if you need to take a minute or two when you first begin working your abs; that's normal. Just begin each set as soon as you're able to. The better shape you're in, the less rest you'll need.

Finally, work to your level. Do the amount and intensity of abdominal training that best suits your current level of fitness.

The Perfect Abdominal Exercises

Beginners should do one or two sets of the following exercises, sticking with the lower end of the recommended range of reps:

- Standing Ab Awareness
- Posture Lifts

- Ab Lifts
- Ball Curls

Once you can do two sets of each exercise easily but with good form, go ahead and increase the number of repetitions per set. When you can do two full sets of the maximum number of repetitions, move on to the intermediate routine.

Intermediates should perform two or three sets of the following exercises, doing somewhere from the middle to the maximum number of recommended repetitions per set.

- Standing Ab Awareness
- Ball Roll-ups
- Posture Lifts
- Slow Bicycles
- Ab Lifts
- Ball Curls

When you can do three sets of each exercise at the top of the repetition range, move on to the advanced routine.

Advanced exercisers should do two or three sets of all ten of the exercises in this chapter and the maximum number of recommended repetitions per set. This should take no more than fifteen minutes to complete once you have an understanding of proper technique.

Regardless of where you start, you should begin to see the fruits of your labor in about four to six weeks. However, let's be clear about what you can expect. If you have a layer of fat over the top of your muscles, no amount of abdominal exercising will define your muscles. Definition is a combination of low body fat and shapely muscles.

Having said that, after a month or so your abs will be significantly stronger, thus your posture will be much improved. And when you can stand up straighter, you look thinner and your middle looks flatter, tighter, and firmer. If you've had back pain, chances are it will be greatly reduced thanks to the balanced support of your middle muscles. You'll probably have more stamina, too, because your lower back won't fatigue as quickly after a day of sitting in your office chair, playing with the kids, or taking a long run.

■ STANDING AB AWARENESS (8–15 REPS)

Muscles Worked: This exercise works all of your core or middle muscles in tandem, much the same way they are used in everyday activities.

Joint Cautions: Mild lower back caution.

Starting Position: Stand tall and relaxed with your feet hip width apart and your arms over your head, palms facing forward. Inhale deeply through your nose. Try to lengthen your torso and pull your belly button inward so the middle of your body feels long and firm.

Exercise: Slowly exhale through your mouth as you lower your arms and pull your ab muscles inward even more. In the final position, your middle will be doubled over slightly and your arms will be at hip level with your palms facing downward. Hold a moment and return to the start.

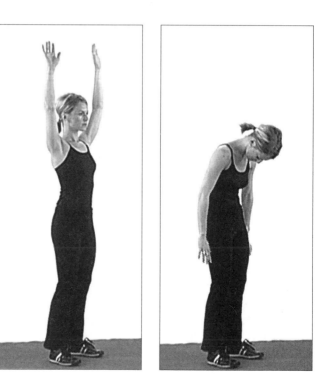

Things to Think About:
- Imagine you are closing a very heavy car trunk. You'll feel a good strong pull through your center as your hands travel downward. This feeling should increase with each repetition.
- Use your abdominals—rather than your arms or hips—to power this small, tight, surprisingly effective movement.

Variations:

- **FOR OBLIQUES:** Lower only one arm down to your side rather than the front.
- **HARDER:** Alternate pulling your arms down one at a time as if you were climbing up a hill.

■ BALL ROLL-UPS (8–15 REPS)

Muscles Worked: This move looks like a crunch but is a lot more focused and effective. It's great for improving spinal flexibility because it teaches you to curl your middle one vertebra at a time.

Joint Cautions: None.

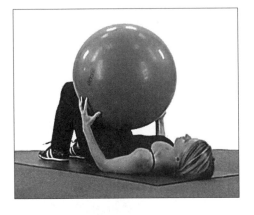

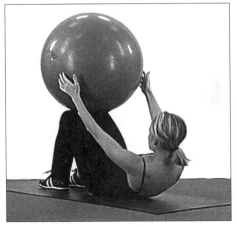

Starting Position: While lying on your back with your knees bent and feet hip width apart, place a physioball on your stomach. Lightly rest your fingertips on both sides of the ball.

Exercise: Inhale and use your fingertips to roll the ball slowly up your thighs to the tops of your knees. As you do this, curl your torso up and forward off the floor. Keep your chin tilted toward your chest and relax your neck. Hold a moment at the top of the movement and slowly roll the ball, and your body, back to the starting position.

Things to Think About:

- Think of your spine as a zipper, slowly unzipping one tooth at a time as you lower yourself and slowly zipping up one tooth at a time to curl back up to the starting position. Your abdominal muscles should feel engaged the entire time.
- Don't rush this exercise. The more slowly and precisely you move, the more effective it will be.

Variations:

- **EASIER:** If you experience any lower-back discomfort or simply feel too weak to complete the entire exercise, roll the ball only halfway up your thighs.
- **HARDER:** At the top of the movement, roll the ball a few inches down your thighs, then back up to the top. Repeat ten times before lowering to the start.

▪ POSTURE LIFTS (8–15 REPS)

Muscles Worked: Teaches your abs and lower back to work in sync with each other. Stretches and strengthens both muscle groups, increases posture awareness, and stretches the backs of your thighs.

Joint Cautions: Mild lower back caution. Keep in mind that the flexibility of Heather, our model, may be greater than yours.

Starting Position: Sit up tall with your legs out in front of you and comfortably apart. Gently flex your feet. Extend your arms out in front of you, shoulders relaxed, palms facing in toward each other. Pull your abs in toward your spine. Inhale deeply through your nose.

Exercise: Exhale through your mouth as you pull your abs inward even more, tuck your chin to your chest, and round forward so that your fingertips move toward your toes. Hold a moment and then straighten up to the starting position so that you are sitting up very tall. Roll up as slowly as possible and hold a moment before moving into the next rep.

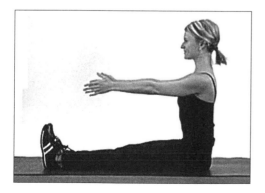 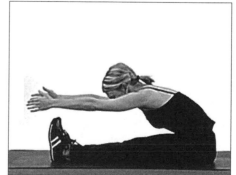

Things to Think About:

- As you lift upward, picture each vertebra stacking directly on top of the one beneath. As you lower, try to move one vertebra at a time. Your abdominals and lower back should feel engaged the entire time, but especially as you lift up tall and pull your muscles inward.

- Focus on keeping your shoulders and neck relaxed as you do this exercise so you can concentrate all of your effort on working the abdominals.

Variations:

- **EASIER:** Bend your knees slightly. This is a good variation if you have poor lower back and hamstring flexibility.

- **HARDER:** As you stretch forward reach your right hand toward your left toe so you get more oblique action. Alternate reps to the right and left.

■ AB PENDULUMS (8–15 REPS EACH SIDE)

Muscles Worked: You'll feel this working your obliques and your rectus abdominis, particularly the lower fibers.

Joint Cautions: Lower back.

Starting Position: Lie on your back with your knees bent and legs held up off the floor directly above your hips. Place your hands behind your head,

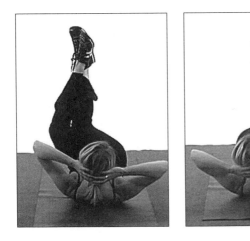

fingertips touching and elbows rounded outward. Curl your head, neck, and shoulders up off the floor. Pull your belly button inward toward the floor.

Exercise: Keeping your upper body still, gently lift your buttocks a small way off the floor and tip your left hip so that your legs sweep a few inches to the left, toward your left elbow. Lower to the starting position and then sweep toward the right. Inhale and exhale once per repetition.

Things to Think About:

- Think of your hips as the pendulum of a clock, ticking slowly and precisely back and forth. You'll feel the muscles at the sides of your waist engage as you lift your legs upward; the more-central muscles will begin to engage as your legs travel past the center and across to the other side.

- Focus on keeping your buttocks just a few inches off the floor as you sweep your legs to the side.

- Maintain a still and stable upper body.

Variations:

- **EASIER:** Keep your upper body down on the floor with your hands along your sides.

- **HARDER:** Instead of returning to the starting position between repetitions, sweep from side to side without allowing your buttocks to touch the floor between reps.

SLOW BICYCLES (8–15 REPS EACH SIDE)

Muscles Worked: Although this exercise zeroes in on your obliques, it gives the other abdominal muscles a good workout, too.

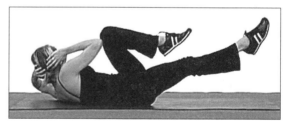

Joint Cautions: Mild neck and lower back caution.

Starting Position: Lie on your back with your left knee bent toward your chest, your right leg extended up off the floor at a 45-degree angle to the floor. Place your hands behind your head, fingertips touching and elbows rounded outward.

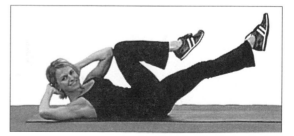

Exercise: Curl your head, neck, and shoulders up off the floor. Rotate from your middle so that your right shoulder is pointing toward your left knee. Hold for a slow count of three, then slowly rotate to the other side by bending your right knee and extending your left leg as your left elbow moves toward your right knee. Again, hold for a slow count of three. Continue rotating to complete reps. Exhale and inhale at least once per twist.

Things to Think About:

- Imagine your abdominals are a wet towel and, as you twist, you are trying to wring all of the water out of the towel. You'll feel a strong pull through your entire middle and spreading out to the sides of your waist, especially as you hold before moving into the next rep.

- Avoid simply moving your elbows toward your knee. Done properly, you should not feel this move in your neck or shoulders at all.

Variations:

- **EASIER:** Hold your extended leg higher than a 45-degree angle to the floor, or reduce the amount of time you hold the twisted position to a slow count of one.

- **HARDER:** Hold your extended leg lower than a 45-degree angle to the floor or extend the amount of time you hold the twisted position to a slow count of five.

AB LIFTS (8–15 REPS)

Muscles Worked: This is an intense move for the entire rectus abdominis muscle, with special emphasis on the lower fibers.

Joint Cautions: Lower back.

Starting Position: Lie on your back with your slightly bent legs held up directly above your hips. Cross your left ankle over your right ankle. Place your hands behind your head, fingertips touching and elbows rounded outward; curl your head, neck, and shoulders up off the floor. Pull your belly button inward toward the floor.

Exercise: Exhale through your mouth and slowly lift your hips and buttocks a small way straight up off the floor. Slowly lower to the start.

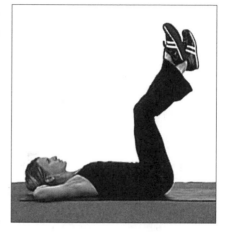

Things to Think About:

- This is a very small, focused movement; imagine your feet are attached to two ropes above you and someone is giving them a small and gentle pull upward to lift your buttocks off the floor. You will feel a strong pull through your middle, especially the area below your belly button.

- Your legs and hips should not roll back toward your nose as you lift your hips up, nor should your upper body move at all during this exercise.

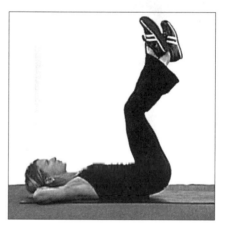

Variations:

- **EASIER:** Keep your upper body on the floor with your arms along your sides.

- **HARDER:** Hold for a slow count of two at the top of the movement before lowering.

■ MINI LEG LOWERS (8–15 REPS)

Muscles Worked: This exercise originates from the lower fibers of the rectus abdominis but works the entire muscle.

Joint Cautions: Strong lower back caution.

Starting Position: Lie on the floor with your hands behind your head; lift your head, neck, and shoulders up off the floor. Raise your legs straight up over your hips. Pull your belly button in toward your spine to anchor your back to the floor.

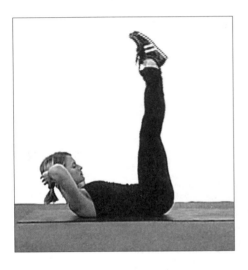

Exercise: Lower your legs toward the floor a very small distance, one or two inches at most. Slowly lift to the start. As you do this exercise, concentrate on keeping your abs tight and your back anchored.

Things to Think About:

- Imagine there is someone standing in front of you, gently pressing your legs to lower them and then releasing them so that they lift back up to the start. You will feel a strong pull through your middle, especially the area below your belly button.
- Do this exercise slowly to make sure you are powering the movement from your abdominal muscles rather than momentum.
- Your hips or buttocks should not rise off the floor at all during this movement, even when you raise your legs back up to the starting position.

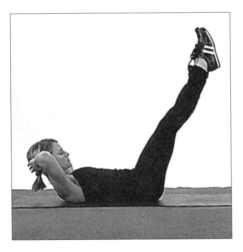

Variations:

- **EASIER:** If holding your legs up straight is too difficult, you may bend your knees slightly.
- **HARDER:** Make a small circle in the air with your feet rather than simply lowering and lifting straight up and down.

▦ HUNDREDS (50–100 PUMPS)

Muscles Worked: This Pilates-inspired movement is an excellent overall abdominal exercise.

Joint Cautions: Lower back.

Starting Position: Lie on your back with your abs pulled inward. Straighten your arms at your sides, holding them a few inches off the floor. Relax your shoulders and bring your knees into your chest; lift your head up and tuck your chin to your chest so that you're looking directly at your navel. Straighten both legs up off the floor and lower them as far as you can while still maintaining contact between your lower back and the floor, but no lower than a 45-degree angle to the floor.

Exercise: Keeping your arms long and extended, pump them vigorously up and down about an inch one hundred times. Inhale every five pumps; exhale every five pumps. Once you have completed the hundred pumps, bend your knees into your chest to rest.

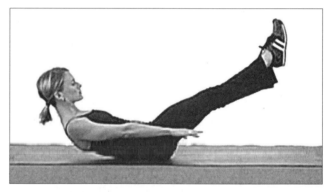

Things to Think About:

- The only thing that should move during this exercise is your arms; concentrate on keeping everything else still and stable. You'll feel a contraction through your entire middle that will gradually intensify through the duration of the exercise.
- It's really important to keep your abdominals pulled inward as you do this exercise.

Variations:

- **EASIER:** Either do this exercise with bent knees or hold your legs up higher than 45 degrees to the floor.
- **HARDER:** Lower your legs so that they are below a 45-degree angle with the floor.

■ HOVER (1–3 REPS)

Muscles Worked: Don't be fooled—this simple exercise is a killer total ab and lower-back move.

Joint Cautions: Lower back, shoulders.

Starting Position: Get down on the floor with your elbows bent and your hands clasped together so that you are balanced on your forearms and undersides of your toes. Tuck your chin in toward your chest. Pull your abs in tight so that your back is straight.

Exercise: Hold this position for a slow count of ten as you breathe slowly and deeply. Focus on keeping your torso straight the entire time. To rest between reps, sit back on your heels and drape your body forward.

Things to Think About:
- Imagine you have a glass of water on your back. You must hold your back flat and still so that the water does not spill. You'll feel a contraction through your entire middle that will gradually intensify through the duration of the exercise.
- Make sure your lower back does not sag downward and your butt does not stick out above the rest of your body.

Variations:
- EASIER: Instead of balancing on your toes, balance on your knees. Shift your body forward in order to lower your torso closer to the floor.
- HARDER: Hold the position for a count of twenty to thirty, or lift one foot a small way off the floor as you maintain the Hover.

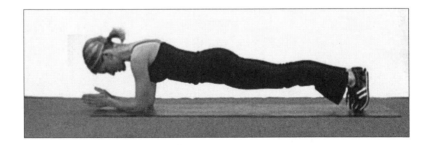

■ BALL CURLS (8–15 REPS)

Muscles Worked: This is one of two moves in this chapter that require the use of a physioball. I've included it because it's an excellent move for both the rectus abdominis and the obliques. It takes a traditional crunch and makes it more effective by forcing your abdominals into a constant contraction in order to prevent rolling off the ball.

Joint Cautions: Lower back, neck.

Starting Position: Sit on top of the center of your physioball with your feet flat on the floor and placed hip width apart. Place your hands behind your head, fingertips touching and elbows rounded outward. Tilt your chin slightly so that there's a few inches of space between your chin and your chest. Gently pull your abdominals inward as you lean back onto the ball so that your entire back, from your tailbone to your shoulders, is resting on the ball. Your head and arms will be suspended above the ball.

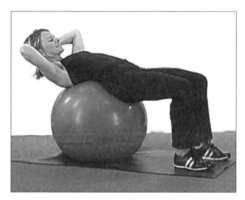

Exercise: Exhale as you curl your head, neck, and shoulders up and forward off the ball. Hold a moment and inhale as you return to the start.

Things to Think About:

- You'll feel a strong contraction throughout your middle, especially as you lift upward.
- Move slowly and carefully to help maintain your balance and reduce any movement other than the crunch.

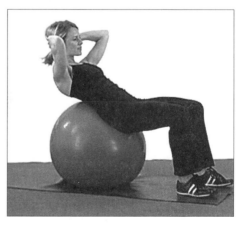

Variations:

- **EASIER:** You can do this curl movement on the floor to eliminate the balance and coordination it takes to stay atop the ball.
- **HARDER:** As you lower, drape your head and shoulders downward on the ball; you'll have to lift up from a lower position, thus making the move more challenging.

The Tenth Month

Grace De Simone, a well-respected personal trainer from New Jersey, has spent a lot of time analyzing the postpartum belly, that abdominal bulge most women experience after they've given birth. She has worked with hundreds of new moms and is a mother of two herself, so she speaks with some authority.

"What I've observed is this—if you had a flat belly before birth, you can attain one again. If you didn't have a flat belly before, what makes you think you are going to have one immediately after the baby is born?" she says.

This is true especially if you develop a condition known as diastasis recti during pregnancy, as many women who have poor abdominal muscle tone do. This is when the edges of the abdominal muscle are separated along the midline because of the increasing pressure from the growing fetus. While not life-threatening, it leaves the tummy soft and poochy, and complications can occur in future pregnancies if the mother does not regain enough abdominal muscle strength and tone.

Even if diastasis recti is not present, De Simone notes that it's an understatement to say that your abdominal area stretches out in the nine months you nurture a child within your belly. When your bundle of joy finally pops out, the skin and underlying muscles do not immediately bounce back into place unless you have some freakishly superhuman genetics, like Cindy Crawford or Madonna.

Achieving your former flatness takes a lot of hard work and, well, time. Most experts say it takes about a year after your baby is born to get your body back to the way it was. "Just remember that muscle work alone is not the answer—you have to burn off fat. That means watching what you eat and getting lots of cardio," De Simone advises.

Banish Belly Bloat

If you're having a bad hair day, you wear a hat. But what about a bad abs day? The kind of day where your middle looks bloated and puffy?

"Younger women often retain water for up to two weeks during their menstrual cycle due to increased estrogen levels," says gynecologist Laura Corio, M.D., author of *The Change Before the Change* (Bantam Dell, 2000).

One way to banish bloat may seem counterintuitive: Drink more water. "Drinking at least eight 8-ounce glasses of water a day acts as a natural diuretic helping to minimize water retention, especially around the belly," Corio states. Other natural diuretics—substances that flush water from your system—include strawberries, grapefruit, and tea.

Avoiding foods and beverages that promote bloat is also a good idea. For instance, overdoing carbonated beverages, raw veggies, beans, and salads can leave you gassy, while salty and highly processed foods pump up water retention due to their high sodium content. One surprise culprit is soup. Corio says that besides packing up to nearly 500 milligrams of sodium per serving, it also gooses up your gaseousness.

6

THE PERFECT LEG AND BUTT WORKOUT

When Celia was growing up in Far Rockaway, New York, she wasn't crazy about having such long legs; kids would call her names like "Giraffa," which means "giraffe" in Spanish. "Once I hit puberty and began playing sports like basketball, I realized legs that long were to my advantage," she says. This part-time model and personal trainer now keeps her legs looking lean and sculpted with regular workouts that include plenty of aerobics and a strength-training routine similar to the one in this chapter. She's happy that her legs and butt have some shape and substance. "I love when women have strong-looking, athletic legs. I think it's sexy," she says.

EXERCISES IN THIS CHAPTER

- Jump Squat Jumps
- Single Leg Squats
- Walking Lunges
- 3-D Lunges
- Side Step-downs
- Dead Lifts
- Calf Presses with Band
- Leg Circles
- Outer Thigh Tosses
- Kick Beats

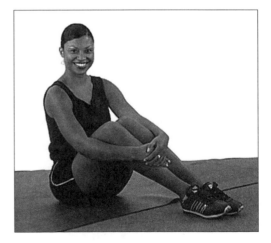

EQUIPMENT NEEDED

Chair or bench

Step

Exercise band

ESTIMATED WORKOUT TIME

- Beginners: 15–20 minutes, two or three times a week
- Intermediates: 20–25 minutes, two or three times a week
- Advanced: 25–30 minutes, two or three times a week

This just in: The miniskirt is back. You can deal with this fashion fact in one of two ways: You can cover your legs, ignore it, and hope it goes away. Or you can put your best leg forward. If you'd like to do the latter, then it's time to shake a leg and get all of those muscles south of the waistline in shape.

Even if the miniskirt goes out of style, showing off your legs is always in fashion one way or another. If they aren't being displayed in a high-cut bathing suit, then it's tight-fitting jeans, short shorts, or sheer fabrics.

I think the pursuit of long, lean, gorgeous legs is practically an obsession for women today. On my iVillage boards I get twenty to thirty questions a week on how to tone some area of the lower body. Not a week goes by that I don't double that number of questions from people I see in the gyms.

A lot of research into what the most effective way to train your legs and butt muscles has found that the best moves are "functional." An exercise is considered functional if it works muscles in a way that closely mirrors how they are normally used in sports and daily activities. Functional exercises don't isolate one muscle group at a time; rather, several muscle groups work in tandem to make the move happen. While all muscles in your body respond very well to functional training, the larger muscles of the buttocks and thighs respond especially well, as do the calf muscles.

Doing functional exercises for the lower half of your body is also important because it can help prevent injuries, especially knee injuries. When you strengthen muscles in the way they're usually used, they're better able to withstand such usage. The moves in this chapter have been selected for their ability not only to shape your legs but also to help you avoid injury.

Actually, you don't really have to remember any fancy buzzwords in order to change the shape of your legs. All you need to know is that the exercises in this chapter have been designed for maximum results. (I can't resist a quick reminder about spot training versus spot reducing here. Remember, you can't eliminate fat from an area of your body by targeting it, but you can change its appearance and shape.) That said, let's run through a quick and easy-to-understand anatomy review of your lower-body muscles to give you better insight into the muscles you'll be working.

Leg and Butt Anatomy Lesson

I've tried to stay away from giving you too many technical terms to think about in this book. Knowing some extravagant Latin name for a muscle isn't going to improve the quality of your workout. However, having some basic knowledge of what you're working can help you zero in on why your workout is structured the way it is and where you should feel each exercise as you're going through your routine. That's why I'd like to explain some general lower-body anatomy to you. I promise I won't load you up with too much unnecessary information, just the facts I think you absolutely need to know.

- **Buttocks.** Also known as the gluteus maximus or the glutes, this is the largest muscle in your body. It spans the entire width of your rear end. It's responsible for all movements that involve sitting, jumping, lifting your leg up high, or pressing it backward. The most effective butt-toning exercises involve bending the knee to 90 degrees and sitting the hips backward and downward.

- **Quadriceps.** This is the group of four muscles that run the length of the front of your thigh. Anytime you straighten your knee from a bent position, your quads get into the act. They're often the main assistance muscles in buttocks exercises, and keeping them strong is essential for preventing knee injuries. I'm not a huge fan of quad isolation exercises, like the leg extension machines you find in many gyms; I think this type of movement places too much force and stress on the knees.

- **Hamstrings.** The hamstrings reside on the opposite side of the joint from the quadriceps, and when they're in shape they give the back of your thigh a nice curvy sweep. The hamstrings assist or are directly involved in many butt moves. Keeping their strength and flexibility balanced with quad strength and flexibility will help prevent knee pain and even hip and lower back pain. The ideal ratio of hamstring to quad strength is 40:60.

- **Inner and Outer Thighs.** These are referred to as the leg adductors and the leg abductors, respectively. The adductors control the movements that involve sweeping one leg in front of the other or when you return your leg from lifting it sideways and upward. The abductors control the movement of your legs that involve lifting your leg up and sideways away from your body. These muscles don't get a lot of usage in modern life, so they tend to respond relatively quickly to targeted strength training.

- **Calves.** The gastrocnemius and the soleus are the two largest muscles in the back of your lower leg. Together they are known as the calf muscles. They power your ankles so you can point and flex your toes. They are among the most oft-used muscle groups in your body because you use them any time you support your body weight, especially during walking and standing. Having strong, shapely calves helps balance the look of the thighs and buttocks. The shape of your calves is largely a matter of genetics. You may have very long calf muscles that run from the back of your knee all the way to your ankles or short muscles that end much higher on the lower leg. Where the muscle attaches will dictate the shape of your calves, although everyone can add contour to their calves.

The Perfect Leg and Butt Exercises

Warm up before you start the Perfect Leg and Butt Workout. Studies show this will enhance your ability to do the exercises properly, and it can help prevent hip, knee, and ankle injuries. The Active-Isolated stretches in chapter 10 are a good warm-up routine. Or you can do five to ten minutes of cycling, brisk walking, or jogging—anything that involves a low-resistance, rhythmic movement of the lower body to increase body temperature and make the muscles more pliable.

Include five to ten minutes of a cool-down that mimics your warm-up after your workout. A cool-down is important to lower muscle temperature and give your body a chance to recover from the workout.

For best results without courting injury or burnout, do this routine two or three times a week. Always give your muscles at least one day of rest in between workouts to allow them time to recover and rebuild.

For a total body-sculpting routine, you can combine this workout with the exercises in "The Perfect Upper Body Workout," chapter 7, and "The Perfect Abdominal Workout," chapter 5. If you have time, you can do all of the exercises on one day, but alternating a day of leg and butt exercises and a day of upper-body and abdominal exercises is also a good way to manage your workouts. Experiment to see what works best for you in terms of preference, scheduling, and results.

Beginners should start with one set of each of the exercises in this chapter. Do ten to fifteen repetitions per set using a weight (or variation of the exercise) that's challenging but not an all-out effort. Rest thirty to ninety seconds between sets. If your goal is to build some strength and stamina in the lower body, you can stick with this routine. If your goal is serious body sculpting or you want to build size and maximum strength, move on to the intermediate routine once you're ready for more.

Intermediate exercisers should do two or three sets of each exercise, eight to fifteen reps per set. Rest thirty to ninety seconds between sets. This is also the routine you should stick with if your goal is body sculpting and developing moderate amounts of strength. If your goal is building size and maximum strength, move on to the advanced routine once you can comfortably complete this one.

Advanced exercisers who are looking to max out size and strength should do three to five sets per exercise, six to eight repetitions per set, using the heaviest weight they can manage while still maintaining good form. Rest for up to three minutes between sets to give your muscles a chance to reboot so they can give it their best effort each and every set.

Whichever routine you perform, do the exercises in the order they're listed. I've set up the routine to work from the largest upper-body muscles to the smallest. This way, the smaller muscles aren't tired out in the earlier stages of the workout and your larger muscles will get a better workout.

You should begin to see results after about six to eight weeks of consistent workouts in the form of a firmer, tighter, and shapelier lower body. If you also watch what you eat and keep up regular cardio workouts to drop body fat, your muscles will begin to take on a more defined appearance. Real strength gains typically come within six weeks of regular training, although you may find yourself able to lift heavier weights after just a couple of workouts. At this point you'll find you have more endurance during activities such as walking, running, climbing stairs, and standing for long periods of time because the lower-body muscles will be in better shape to offer support. You may also find that any knee, hip, or ankle soreness will be diminished as a result of stronger muscles helping to stabilize and support the joints.

JUMP SQUAT JUMPS

Muscles Worked: This exercise targets just about every muscle south of the belly button, including your buttocks, the front and back of thighs, the inner and outer thighs, and the calves.

Joint Cautions: Knees, lower back.

Starting Position: Stand tall with your feet hip width apart, toes angled slightly outward, and your hands on your hips. Pull your abs in and bend your knees slightly.

Exercise: Bend your knees until your thighs are parallel to the floor. As you stand up, jump a few inches into the air and land softly with your

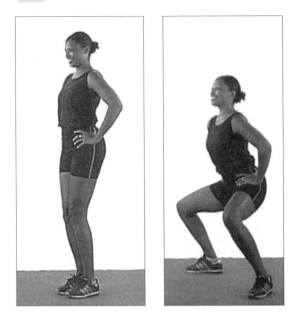

feet a few inches wider than hip width apart. Squat down again and as you stand up, jump back to the starting position.

Things to Think About:

- As you do the exercise, imagine you're going for a basketball jump shot. You'll feel all of your leg muscles working, especially as you jump upward and as you bend into the squat.
- Take care to land softly and make sure that your knees never shoot past your toes.
- Keep your upper body as straight as possible. Don't allow yourself to fold too far forward; this may mean you can't bend your knees until your thighs are parallel to the floor, but that's okay.

Variations:

- **EASIER:** Do the basic squat as described on page 254.
- **HARDER:** Hold a dumbbell in each hand with your arms down at your sides.

SINGLE LEG SQUATS

Muscles Worked: This exercise does an excellent job of isolating your buttocks, hip, and thigh muscles.

Joint Cautions: Knees.

Starting Position: Stand tall about a stride's length in front of a chair or a bench. With the top of your right foot facing down toward the floor, prop that foot up on the bench and bend your right leg a few inches. Place your hands on your hips or keep them down at your sides, whichever is most comfortable. Pull your abs inward.

Exercise: Bend your left knee to lower your upper body toward the floor. When your left thigh is parallel to the floor, stand back up to the starting position. Complete all reps and switch to the other side.

Things to Think About:

- You'll feel your front thigh working the entire time, but especially when you stand back up. You'll also feel a stretch through your back inner thigh as you squat.
- Your back knee may or may not bend as you move through the exercise depending on your positioning and your flexibility.
- Resist leaning your upper body too far forward, and avoid allowing your front knee to move forward of your toes.

Variations:

- **EASIER:** Rather than placing your foot up on a bench, place one leg out in front of you and lift your heel up. Bend your hip and back knee until your thigh is parallel to the floor or as much as you can comfortably bend.
- **HARDER:** Hold a dumbbell in each hand to add resistance.

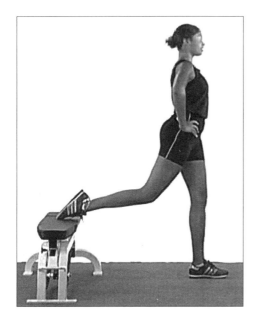 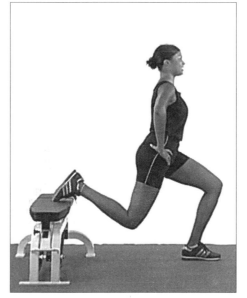

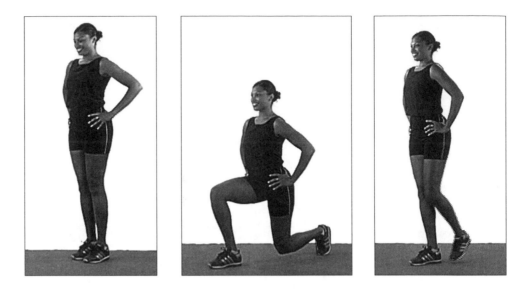

■ WALKING LUNGES

Muscles Worked: This super-intense exercise targets your buttocks, thighs, and calves.

Joint Cautions: Knees, lower back.

Starting Position: Stand tall with your feet hip width apart with your hands on your hips. Pull your abs inward.

Exercise: Step your right leg forward a natural stride's length. As your right foot makes contact with the floor, bend both of your knees until your right thigh is parallel to the floor and your left thigh is perpendicular to it. Stand back up to the start, bringing your left foot forward to your right foot. Next, perform a lunge by stepping your left foot forward. As you alternate lunges you will travel around the room.

Things to Think About:
- Pretend you're walking on a sidewalk full of cracks you don't want to step on.
- You will feel a contraction in your front thigh as you stand up, and a stretch through your back leg as you step forward and bend your knees.

Variations:

- **EASIER:** Perform a stationary lunge as described on page 255.
- **HARDER:** Don't come back to the center between repetitions. Instead, move forward in an exaggerated walk. You can also swing your arms forcefully to help power the movement.

3-D LUNGES

Muscles Worked: This exercise challenges all of your lower-body muscles and is also great for developing a sense of balance and coordination.

Joint Cautions: Knees, lower back.

Starting Position: Stand tall with your feet hip width apart, your hands on your hips, and your abs contracted.

Exercise: Step forward with your right foot a comfortable stride's length and bend both of your knees until your right thigh is parallel to the floor and your left leg is perpendicular to it. Stand back up to the start and then lunge your right leg to the side so that your right leg bends and your left leg straightens. Stand back up to the starting position. Finally, lunge your right leg back behind you a comfortable distance, bending your knees

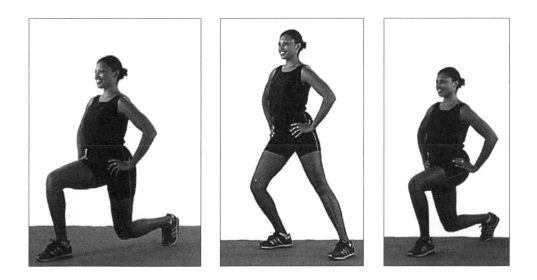

until your left thigh is parallel to the floor and your right thigh is perpendicular to it. Stand back up once more and repeat the entire sequence, leading with your left leg.

Things to Think About:

- Think of your lead leg as the little hand of a clock, and lunge to 12:00, 3:00, and 6:00. You will feel both legs working throughout the entire exercise, but you'll feel the strongest contraction through the front of the thigh of your lead leg every time you stand back up to the starting position.
- Move slowly to maintain your balance.
- Avoid allowing your knees to travel out in front of your toes.

Variations:

- **EASIER:** Hold on to a sturdy object for support during the front and back lunge portion of this exercise. You may also consider having someone spot you to help you with your balance.
- **HARDER:** Add several additional lunge positions, lunging to 1:00 and 2:00 as well.

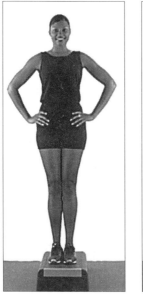
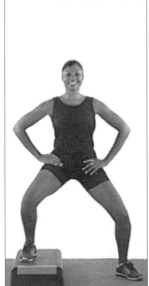

■ SIDE STEP-DOWNS

Muscles Worked: An intense exercise that strengthens all of the muscles in your buttocks and thighs, with special emphasis on your inner and outer thighs.

Joint Cautions: Knees.

Starting Position: Stand tall in the center of a low step platform with your hands on your hips and your abs contracted.

Exercise: Step off the side of the platform with your left foot. As your foot touches the floor, bend both knees about six inches. Press off the ball of your left foot to lightly spring back to the starting position. Complete all reps with your right foot and then repeat on the left.

Things to Think About:
- You will feel the inner thighs of both legs stretching and working as you step out to the side, and you will feel both thighs—but especially your lead leg—as you step back to the starting position.
- Focus on keeping your upper body upright and straight rather than allowing it to fold forward.

Variations:
- **EASIER:** Do the same exercise on the floor.
- **HARDER:** Alternate left and right step-downs doing a low hop across the center of the platform between reps.

DEAD LIFTS

Muscles Worked: An excellent hamstring, buttocks, and lower-back toner.

Joint Cautions: Lower back.

Starting Position: Hold a dumbbell in each hand with your arms down at your sides and your palms facing back behind you. Stand tall with your knees straight and your abdominals pulled inward.

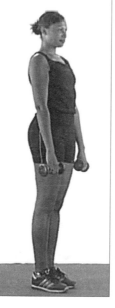
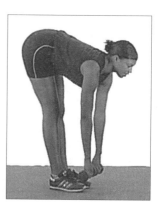

Exercise: Keeping your knees straight, lean forward from your hips until your upper body is as close to perpendicular to the floor as your flexibility allows and your arms are hanging down in front of you. Stand back up to the start.

Things to Think About:

- This exercise mimics picking up something heavy off the floor. You'll feel this exercise in the backs of your thighs and your lower back as you stand back up to the starting position.

Variations:

- **EASIER:** Bend your knees slightly. This is a good version to do if you're prone to lower back troubles.
- **HARDER:** Hold a straight bar instead of two dumbbells.

■ CALF PRESSES WITH BAND

Muscles Worked: A great calf and shin move.

Joint Cautions: Mild ankle caution.

Starting Position: Sit in a chair or on the floor with an exercise band wrapped securely around the instep of your right foot and your right leg out straight. Hold one end of the band in each hand and pull tight enough to create tension in the band. You can bend your left knee or position it however you feel comfortable.

Exercise: Point your toes forward, tightening the resistance as you go. Hold a moment at the top of the movement and then flex your foot, moving past the starting position, pulling on the band to assist you. Complete all reps and repeat with your left foot.

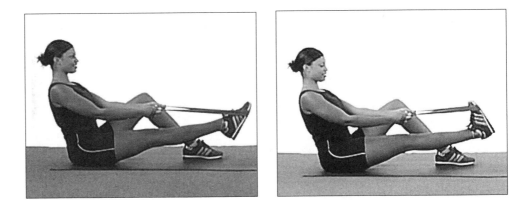

Things to Think About:

- You'll feel a strong contraction in your calf as you point your foot and a strong stretch as you flex it.
- Keep your foot moving in a straight line rather than allowing it to turn inward or outward.

Variations:

- **EASIER:** Use a towel instead of a band. The resistance, or tension, won't be as intense.
- **HARDER:** Use a thicker rubber band, which creates more resistance.

◼ LEG CIRCLES

Muscles Worked: Your entire thigh works during this move, but especially your inner and outer thighs. This is also a hip and thigh flexibility booster.

Joint Cautions: Hips, lower back.

Starting Position: Lie on your back with your abs contracted and your arms along your sides. Bend your left knee so that your left foot is flat on the floor and extend your right leg straight up, parallel to the floor if your flexibility allows. Softly point your right toe.

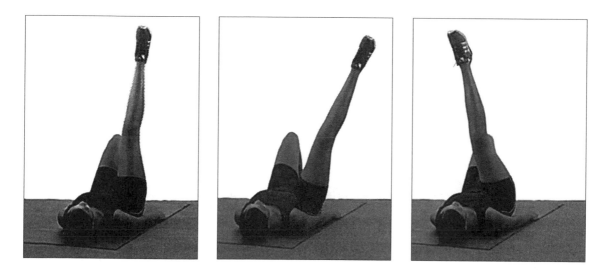

Exercise: Keeping your leg as fully lengthened as possible, move your right leg in a small clockwise circle ten times and then ten times in a counterclockwise circle. Repeat with your left leg.

Things to Think About:
- Imagine you are drawing a circle about the size of a dinner plate on the ceiling with your toes. You will feel this exercise in your hips and the very top of the front of your thighs. You will also feel a contraction in your inner thighs as your leg moves toward the midline of your body. You may also feel this exercise in your abs, especially if you focus on keeping them contracted.
- Focus on keeping your abs pulled in and every part of your body still except for your working leg.
- Keep your shoulders down and relaxed.

Variations:
- **EASIER:** Bend your working knee slightly or hold your leg closer to the floor.
- **HARDER:** Draw bigger circles, placing emphasis on extending your leg lower as you move it across your body.

■ OUTER THIGH TOSSES

Muscles Worked: This exercise isolates the outer thigh muscles and also targets the buttocks and inner thighs.

Joint Cautions: None. Keep in mind your flexibility may not be as great as that of our model, Celia.

Starting Position: Lie on your left side with your legs slightly forward of your body, one hip stacked directly on top of the other. Turn your right leg out slightly so that your knee is facing the ceiling, and flex your foot. Rest your head on your outstretched arm or in your left hand, whichever is more comfortable. Place your right hand in front of your chest for support.

Exercise: Using control, toss your right leg up as high as it will go. Point your toes and then lower to the start, creating resistance by tightening your buttocks muscles and lengthening your leg as much as possible. Flex your foot again before moving into the next rep. After ten reps, repeat the movement starting with your toes pointed and then flexing as you move back to the start. Complete all reps and repeat with your left leg.

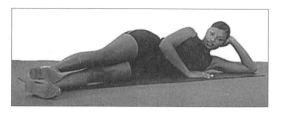

Things to Think About:

• Imagine you are pressing a heavy object down with the inner part of your thigh as you lower your leg. You'll feel this exercise through the center of your buttocks, the outer edges of your hips, and your inner thighs as you press downward.

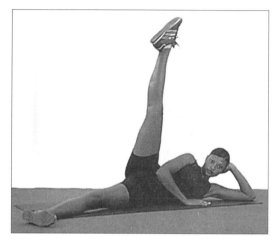

Variations:

• **EASIER:** Bend your knees slightly.
• **HARDER:** Each time you lower your leg, alternate placing your foot a little behind you and a little in front of you.

KICK BEATS

Muscles Worked: This unusual exercise is deceptively simple but is a killer buttocks and back-of-thigh shaping exercise.

Joint Cautions: Mild lower back caution.

Starting Position: Lie on your stomach with your forehead resting on the backs of your folded hands. Extend your legs out straight and pull your abs up and in as if you're trying to create a space between your belly button and the floor.

Exercise: Flex your feet and lift your legs a few inches off the floor. In a quick, controlled motion, beat your heels together ten times. Lower to the starting position. This is one repetition.

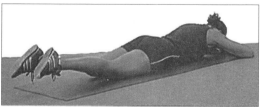

Things to Think About:

- This movement is like clapping your hands together quickly—but with your feet! It will feel awkward at first but gets easier every time you do it. You'll feel a contraction through your buttocks and inner thighs the entire time your legs are lifted.

Variations:

- **EASIER:** Place a pillow or towel under your hips.
- **HARDER:** Increase the number of beats per repetition to twenty.

Revving Up Your Rear View

Working with weights is a great way to sculpt the lower body. Adding endurance activities that place a lot of emphasis can speed up the toning process. The following aerobic workouts work all of your hip and thigh muscles but place special emphasis on specific areas. (Please remember: These activities will tone, not bulk.)

- **Butt**
  - Walking hills, walking on an incline on the treadmill
  - Climbing stairs, stair-climbing machines (especially rolling staircases)
  - Recumbent bike
  - Step aerobics

- **Quads**
  - Upright bike, outdoor cycling, spinning
  - Elliptical trainer
  - Walking and running on the flat
  - Kickboxing

- **Hamstrings**
  - Sprinting
  - Swimming with the butterfly or breast stroke using a double leg kick
  - Rowing
  - Pilates, yoga

- **Inner and Outer Thighs**
  - Ice skating

- In-line skating
- Soccer
- Dance

- **Calves**
  - Jumping rope
  - Long-distance walking and running
  - Basketball
  - Volleyball

Illegitimate Leg Lore

Here are some lower-body training myths that don't have a leg to stand on.

- **The more reps the better.** More is not necessarily better. Sometimes it's just more. High-rep, low-weight exercises such as leg lifts, even if you do a hundred of them, are ineffective because they don't work the muscles hard enough to get results.

- **You can spot-reduce.** Yes, you can change the shape of a muscle with spot training, but you can never spot-reduce. No amount of lower-body training will melt fat off your hips or reduce the size of your butt unless you diminish the overlying body fat from those areas. The only way to do this is by eating fewer calories and burning them with cardiovascular exercise.

- **Weight training makes you bulky.** Many women are afraid weight training will bulk up their legs. In most cases this is simply not true. Doing relatively few sets where you give a good effort will tone and strengthen your muscles, but it's not likely to add much size. Very few women have the genetics to build massive tree-trunk legs unless they spend hours in the gym and possess (or take) an unusually high amount of male hormones.

- **Lower-body training is all you need.** Even if your only goal is to improve the appearance of your lower half, don't skimp on upper-body training. An in-shape upper body makes your lower body look smaller and gives it a more balanced and better-proportioned appearance.

Cellulite

Although we've given it its own identity, cellulite doesn't really differ from any other type of body fat except that it's laced together with connective tissue called collagen. The fat pokes through spaces in the collagen, producing a puckery, dimply appearance—usually on the rear and thighs—that we've come to know and loathe. Women are more susceptible to cellulite because we hold more body fat in our lower bodies than men do. We also have hormones that seem to promote the appearance of cellulite, which is why even thin women can have a little "cottage cheese."

Hucksters have made a fortune selling us pills, potions, and wraps that they claim will banish cellulite. There's even a seaweed soap that's being sold at a brisk pace by health food stores and via the Internet that promises to wash cellulite away. These products include gingko biloba, sweet clover, grape-seed bioflavonoids, dried *Fucus vesiculosus* (a kelplike seaweed found off the Atlantic coast of Europe), and a host of other "active" ingredients with tongue-twisting names. They profess to eliminate cellulite by increasing blood circulation, reducing fluid buildup, stimulating metabolism, "freeing" trapped fat, and killing "fat storage receptors."

Come on, now! We should know better than to buy into this unsubstantiated, made-up pseudoscientific mumbo jumbo. No legitimate research exists to show that any of these products has even the slightest effect on cellulite.

So is there a way to banish the bumpiness and clumpiness? You deal with cellulite the same way you deal with any body fat: by eating a healthy diet and doing regular exercise. There are also some over-the-counter firming creams on the market that do offer marginal and temporary improvements. However, those ripples can hold on stubbornly and may be impossible to completely diminish without plastic surgery.

7

THE PERFECT UPPER-BODY WORKOUT

As someone who is naturally long and lean, Gina has had to make an extra effort to work on her upper-body strength. She does this with two or three weight sessions a week that are similar to the routine in this chapter—and lots of yoga. "I'm stronger and more self-confident in my thirties than I was in my twenties," she says. Recently, when Gina was redecorating her apartment, she had to walk several blocks and up several flights of stairs with a rolled-up carpet over one shoulder and a heavy box in the other hand. "It was no big deal," she says nonchalantly. And now that her upper body is so buff and beautiful, her favorite thing to do at parties is to make a muscle and have people feel how firm her arms are. "It's very impressive," she says. "I get a lot of attention for having such a thin yet strong frame—especially from men."

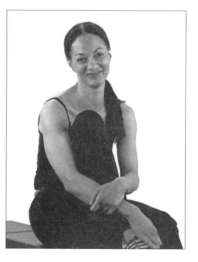

EXERCISES IN THIS CHAPTER

- Chest Flys
- Dumbbell Pullovers
- Incline Dumbbell Presses
- Dumbbell Rows

- Gladiator Pulls with Band
- Lateral Raises
- Back Delt Flys
- Concentration Curls
- Lying Kick-outs
- Wrist Curls

EQUIPMENT NEEDED

- Two to five sets of dumbbells
- A sturdy, stable chair or workout bench
- An exercise band

ESTIMATED WORKOUT TIME

- Beginners: 15–20 minutes, two or three times a week
- Intermediates: 25–35 minutes, two or three times a week
- Advanced: 35–45 minutes, two or three times a week

Madonna. Janet Jackson. Buffy the Vampire Slayer. Xena the Warrior Princess. All these women are beauty role models with one thing in common: killer upper bodies.

This is big news. Women have never considered having a great upper body something to strive for. Oh, sure, you might yearn for a certain amount of cleavage, but most women haven't traditionally put having a broad back or sculpted shoulders at the top of their wish lists.

I realized there had been a shift in thinking when a few months ago I heard Joan and Melissa Rivers dishing about bodies of the rich and famous on their E! show and referring to the well-toned upper body as "the perfect summer accessory, something no best-dressed woman should be without." Okay, so maybe Joan and Melissa aren't exactly a litmus test for anything, but in this instance I think they're on to something.

Women are usually most dissatisfied with the shape of their hips, butt, and thighs and concentrate the bulk of their efforts on these areas. I agree that it's essential to work the lower body, but that's only half the picture.

Nikki is one of my iVillage readers whom I bugged for months to do some upper-body training even though she told me her goal was strictly lower-body toning. "For many years I only did toning exercises for my legs and rear but could never escape the feeling that I looked out of proportion. When I finally started doing upper-body training, I saw a dramatic change in my appearance. I finally have a body that looks balanced," she admits.

Working your upper body gives you a little extra width across the top. Many women hear the words "extra width" and think, "No, thanks!" But in this case it's a good thing. By slightly broadening your top half, you give the illusion that your bottom half is smaller even if you don't shrink an inch in your hips or butt. (And if you do, so much the better.) Your waist will appear smaller, too, because it *is* smaller in relation to your shoulders and back. It's all about creating proportion, symmetry, and balance.

A strong upper body is also important for good posture. Strong back and shoulder muscles keep you from looking round-shouldered and pulled forward; strong chest muscles help you hold yourself upright and lifted. As you get older, weight training will help preserve bone density in the upper body so you don't develop a hunched-over look.

Fortunately, a better-toned upper half is usually an attainable goal. Upper-body muscles often respond quickly to weight training because they're starved for attention. Most women don't use the muscles north of their waistline very much in everyday life.

Upper-Body Anatomy Lesson

Before we get into the nitty-gritty workout details, I'd like to give you a simple anatomy lesson featuring the main muscles of your upper body. As much as I hate to get mired in technical jargon, I do think it's important to have some basic knowledge of what muscles you're working and why you're working them. I promise you this information will come in handy. It will help you zero in on where you should feel each exercise and clue you in to the type of result you can expect. This is by no means a complete graduate-level explanation of upper-body anatomy, but it's probably all the information you absolutely need to know.

- **Upper back muscles.** These muscles are the centerpiece of a beautifully toned upper body. Along with the shoulders, they create a desirable V-shaped physique that makes your hips and waist look smaller. When toned, these muscles help you pull off low-backed, strapless, and spaghetti-strap styles with confidence. The main upper back muscles you need to know about are the latissimus dorsi (lats); they form the wings, the outer edges of your back. They are the largest muscle in your upper body and run from the center of your mid-lower back all the way into your armpits. All upper back muscles are involved in pulling movements.

- **Chest muscles.** The next largest upper-body muscles, the pectorals (pecs), are responsible for all pushing movements. Since they reside directly under your breasts, keeping them toned and strong is the secret to keeping your breasts looking firm and young.

- **Shoulders.** The shoulder is a four-headed muscle known in technical terms as the deltoids or delts. It caps the front, top, and sides of your arm and upper back. Shapely shoulders make you appear leaner because they balance out the lower half of your body. Since the shoulders are involved in virtually every upper-body movement in one way or another, it's important to work them so that all of your upper-body movements are strong.

- **Rotator cuff.** I've included the rotator cuff, the four-muscle structure that integrates with the upper back and shoulders, in this discussion not because it makes a particular contribution to your upper body's appearance but because it is a very commonly injured area. Most shoulder pain is really rotator cuff pain. Anyone who is serious about strength training has got to pay attention to the strength and health of this small but significant muscle group. That's why several exercises in this chapter are at least partially aimed at working the rotator cuff.

- **Triceps.** The triceps muscles, which run the length of the back of your arm, are the bane of many women's existence. You've probably heard one of the many nicknames for this area: the flapping clothesline, bingo arms, the Hadassah hang, and Hi Janes. Because this muscle gets almost no use in the life of an average woman, it often develops a loose, flabby quality even when there isn't a lot of excess fat stored in this area. The good news here is that this is a muscle that responds quickly to weight training—it's involved in any exercise that calls for straightening the arms and pushing—so you are likely to see dramatic improvements in a relatively short period of time. Strengthening this muscle also helps alleviate tennis elbow and other repetitive-movement injuries.

- **Biceps.** Biceps reside on the opposite side of the upper arm from the triceps. They bend the arms and assist the back and shoulders with pushing movements. Toning them—along with the triceps—makes wearing sleeveless and short-sleeved styles a happier experience. Like the triceps, this muscle responds rapidly to strength training, and strengthening it can help ease repetitive-movement injuries.

- **Forearms.** While no one is writing love songs about the forearms, they're still a pretty important collection of muscles. They're involved in gripping, typing, holding—anytime you use your hands and fingers. Better grip strength allows you to lift more weight when working other muscles, plus you'll be less likely to develop carpal tunnel syndrome and other types of repetitive-movement injuries.

The Perfect Upper-Body Exercises

With any type of strength training, it's important to warm up before you start, and the Perfect Upper-Body Workout is no exception. The Active-Isolated stretches in chapter 10 can serve as a suitable warm-up, as can five to ten minutes of a cardio activity such as using a bike with moving arm attachments, rowing, jumping rope, or using a cross-country ski machine—anything that involves a low-resistance, rhythmic movement of the upper body to increase body temperature and make the muscles more pliable and ready for work. If you work out in a gym that has something called an upper-body bicycle, this is an excellent warm-up for upper-body weight lifting as well.

For best results without courting injury or burnout, do this routine two or three times a week. Always give your muscles at least one day of rest in between workouts to allow them time to recover and rebuild.

For a total body-sculpting routine, you can combine this workout with the Perfect Leg and Butt Workout (chapter 6) and the Perfect Abdominal Workout (chapter 5). If you have time, you can do all of the exercises on one day, but alternating a day of upper-body exercises with a day of lower-body and abdominal exercises is also a good way to manage your workouts. Experiment to see what works best for you in terms of preference, scheduling, and results.

Beginners whose main goal is to build some strength and tone should do one set of each exercise, twelve to fifteen repetitions per set, using a weight that's challenging but not the maximum you can lift. Rest thirty to ninety seconds between sets. If you're aiming for serious body sculpting or trying to build size and maximum strength, move on to the intermediate routine once you're ready for more.

Intermediate exercisers should do two or three sets of each exercise, eight to fifteen reps per set. Rest thirty to ninety seconds between sets. This is also the routine you should stick with if your goal is body sculpting and developing moderate amounts of strength. If your goal is building size and serious strength, move on to the advanced routine once you can breeze through the intermediate routine.

Advanced exercisers who are looking to max out size and strength should do three to five sets per exercise, six to eight repetitions per set, using the heaviest weight they can manage while still maintaining good form. Rest for up to three minutes between sets to give your muscles a chance to fully recover so they can get ready to give it their best effort in each and every set.

Whichever level you're at, do the exercises in the order in which they're listed. I've set up the routine to work from the largest upper-body muscles to the smallest. This way, the smaller muscles aren't tired out in the earlier stages of the workout and your larger muscles will get a better workout.

The reason for this is that all exercises, even if they do a decent job of isolating a particular muscle, rely on many muscles to perform movement. The smaller muscles of the biceps, for instance, assist the larger muscles of the upper back to pull your arm upward during the Dumbbell Row. If you were to do your curls first and exhaust your biceps, you wouldn't be able to lift as much weight for as many reps of the Dumbbell Row, so your upper-back muscles would get short shrift.

You should begin to see the fruits of your labor after about three to six weeks of consistent workouts. You'll notice that your muscles look firmer, tighter, and shapelier. Women have also told me that their bust looks higher (as in moving in the opposite direction of gravity) after a few weeks of training. As I've said previously in this chapter, women's upper-body muscles tend to respond well to weight training, since they're typically so underutilized in everyday activities. If you also watch what you eat and keep up regular cardio workouts to drop body fat, your muscles will begin to take on a more defined appearance. Real strength gains typically come within six weeks of beginning regular training, although you may find yourself able to lift heavier weights after just a couple of workouts.

■ CHEST FLYS

Muscles Worked: Your chest, shoulders, and triceps get an excellent workout with this exercise.

Joint Cautions: Shoulders, rotator cuff, elbows.

Starting Position: Lie on a weight bench with a dumbbell in each hand and place your feet flat on the floor (or up on the bench if it's more comfortable). Straighten your arms upward so that they are directly over your shoulders and your palms face in toward each other, wrists straight. Pull your abdominals in.

Exercise: In an arclike path, bend your elbows and lower your arms down and out to the sides until your elbows are just below shoulder level. Straighten your arms back up to the starting position.

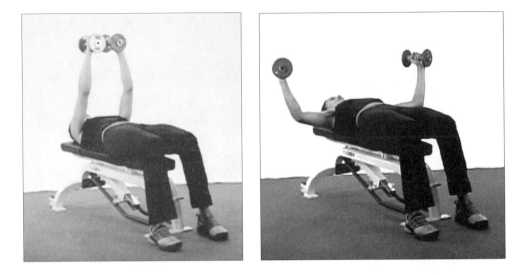

Things to Think About:

- In the lowermost position your arms will form a shallow W. You'll feel a pull or contraction through the outer edges of your chest, the center of your shoulders, and the backs of your arms as you straighten your arms. Near the end of the set, the contraction may spread toward the center of the chest.

- Avoid lowering your arms any lower than described; this can place undue strain on the rotator cuff.

- Keep your abs pulled inward so you don't arch your back.

Variations:

- **EASIER:** Perform this exercise on the floor rather than a bench.

- **HARDER:** Incline the bench to about 30 degrees. You'll feel this more in your upper chest.

■ DUMBBELL PULLOVERS

Muscles Worked: This super-efficient exercise strengthens the upper back, chest, shoulders, arms, and abs.

Joint Cautions: Shoulders, rotator cuff, elbows.

Starting Position: Holding a single dumbbell with both hands, lie on the bench with your feet flat on the floor and your arms directly over your shoulders. Turn your palms up so that one end of the dumbbell is resting in the gap between your palms and the other end is hanging down over your face. Pull your abdominals in.

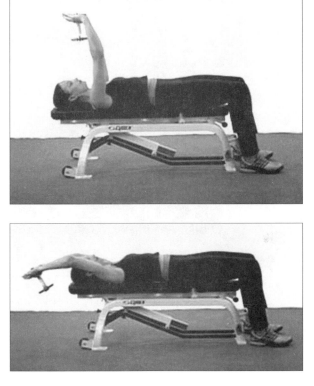

Exercise: In an arclike path, lower the dumbbell back and behind you until the bottom head of the dumbbell is level with the back of your head. Lift back up to the starting position.

Things to Think About:

- You'll feel a stretch through your chest and rib cage as you lower the weight and a contraction along the outer edges of your back and through your arms as you lift up.
- Avoid arching your back off the bench, especially as you lower the weight.
- Don't bend your elbows to lower the weight; this movement is powered from the shoulder joint.

Variations:

- EASIER: Do this exercise on the floor.
- HARDER: Rather than lying on the bench, prop your upper back along the edge of the bench with your feet hip width apart and flat on the floor. As you lower the weight, it will move down and over the bench to the other side.

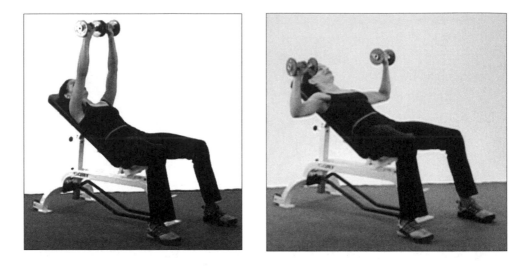

■ INCLINE DUMBBELL PRESSES

Muscles Worked: Your chest, shoulders, and triceps get a workout with this exercise.

Joint Cautions: Shoulders, rotator cuff.

Starting Position: Angle the back of a weight bench to about 30 degrees. Lie on the weight bench with a dumbbell in each hand and place your feet flat on the floor (or up on the bench if it's more comfortable). Straighten your arms upward so that they are directly over your shoulders, with your palms face forward and your wrists straight. Pull your abdominals in.

Exercise: Bend your elbows to lower the weights. When your elbows are just below shoulder level, straighten your arms back up to the starting position.

Things to Think About:
- You'll feel this exercise through the outer edges of your upper chest as well as the center of your shoulders and backs of your arms as you lift the weights.
- Avoid arching your back to lift the weight.
- Try not to bend your arms any further than directed, as this can be very stressful to your shoulders and rotator cuff.

Variations:
- **EASIER:** Perform this same exercise on a flat bench or while lying on the floor.
- **HARDER:** Raise the back of the bench 1–3 positions and perform an incline fly exercise.

■ DUMBBELL ROWS

Muscles Worked: This exercise targets your upper back, shoulders, and biceps.

Joint Cautions: Shoulders, lower back.

Starting Position: Stand to the left of your weight bench and hold a dumbbell in your left hand with your palm facing in. Pull your abdominals in and bend forward from your hips so that your back is parallel, or slightly above parallel, to the floor. Bend knees slightly. Place your right hand on top of the bench for support and let your left arm hang down.

Exercise: Bend your elbow to lift your arm up. When your elbow is just above waist level, slowly straighten your arm back to the starting position. Complete all reps and then repeat with the right arm.

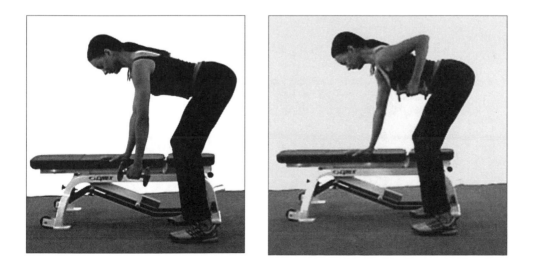

Things to Think About:

- This exercise resembles pulling the start cord of a lawn mower. You'll feel a strong contraction through the outer edges of your upper back and in the front of your arms as you lift the weight. You may also feel your shoulder muscles working.
- Keep your abdominals contracted so that your back remains naturally arched.
- Squeeze your shoulder blades together as you lift the weight; this will work more surface area of your back muscles.

Variations:

- **EASIER:** Put your right knee up on the bench for support.
- **HARDER:** Try the Bar Rows version described on page 163.

■ GLADIATOR PULLS WITH BAND

Muscles Worked: This exercise targets the entire shoulder area, especially the back of the shoulder and rotator cuff.

Joint Cautions: Mild rotator cuff caution.

Starting Position: Kneel with your left foot in front of your right foot, one end of an exercise band anchored under your left foot. Keep your spine

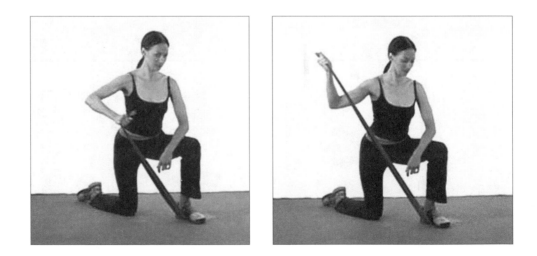

tall, tighten your abs, and grasp the other end of the band in your right hand. Place your left forearm on your left thigh for support.

Exercise: Shift your weight back slightly as you raise your right arm so that your elbow is at shoulder level and your hand is slightly behind your head. Slowly and with control return to the starting position. Complete all reps and repeat with the left arm.

Things to Think About:
- Focus on powering the movement from the rotation of your shoulder. You'll feel a strong contraction deep in the center and back of your shoulder as you lift up.
- Control the band on both the way up and the way down. Moving too fast increases your risk of injury.

Variations:
- **EASIER:** Do this movement while sitting in a chair or on a weight bench.
- **HARDER:** At the top of the movement, press your hand backward eight to ten times in a pulsing movement before lowering to the starting position.

LATERAL RAISES

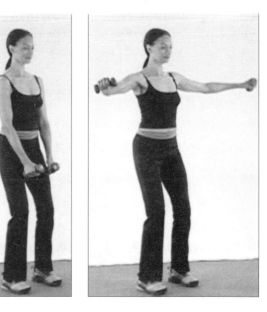

Muscles Worked: A great shoulder toner.

Joint Cautions: Rotator cuff.

Starting Position: Hold a dumbbell in each hand and stand up tall with your feet hip width apart. Bend your elbows slightly, turn your palms toward each other, and bring your hands together so that the dumbbells are touching and level with the front of the tops of your thighs. Pull your abdominals in.

Exercise: Raise your arms up and out to the sides until your hands are level with your shoulders. Keep your arms and hands a few inches in front of your body and shoulders. Slowly lower to the starting position.

Things to Think About:
- This movement always reminds me of pouring two pitchers of water. You'll feel a strong contraction on the sides and middle of your shoulders as you lift.
- Maintain that slight bend in your elbows throughout.
- There's no need to lift the weights any higher than shoulder level.

Variations:
- **EASIER:** Bend your arms even more to take the pressure off your shoulders and rotator cuff.
- **HARDER:** Try this exercise seated instead of standing.

■ BACK DELT FLYS

Muscles Worked: An essential exercise for strengthening and toning your upper back and back-of-shoulder muscles.

Joint Cautions: Shoulders, rotator cuff, lower back.

Starting Position: Hold a dumbbell in each hand and sit on the edge of the bench. Lean forward from your hips so that your upper back is straight and slightly above parallel to the floor. Stretch your arms down so that your palms are facing each other, with the weights behind your calves and directly under your knees. Pull your abdominals in.

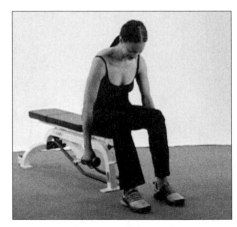
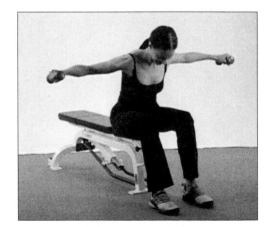

Exercise: Keeping a slight bend in your elbows, lift your arms up and out to the sides until your hands are level with your shoulders. Slowly lower to the starting position.

Things to Think About:
- Imagine you are scooping a large pile of clothing off the floor. You'll feel a strong tension though the back and center of your shoulders as you lift.
- Squeeze your shoulder blades together as you lift the weight.
- Don't round your back; keep it naturally flat.

Variations:
- **EASIER:** Do this exercise from a standing position, leaning forward at a 45-degree angle from your hips.
- **HARDER:** Rotate your hands so that your palms are facing backward.

■ CONCENTRATION CURLS

Muscles Worked: This exercise zeroes in on the biceps muscles.

Joint Cautions: Slight elbow caution.

Starting Position. Hold a dumbbell in your right hand and sit on the edge of a bench or a chair with your feet slightly wider than hip width apart. Lean forward from your hips and place your right elbow against the inside of your right thigh, just behind your knee. Allow the weight to hang down near the inside of your ankle. Place your left palm on top of your left thigh.

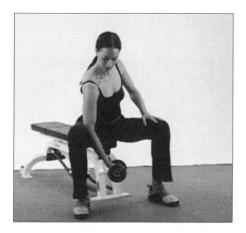 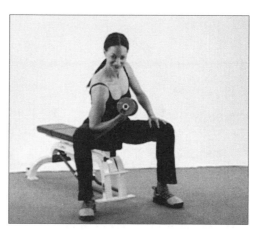

Exercise: Bend your elbow and curl the weight up to shoulder level. Slowly lower to the starting position. Complete all reps and repeat with your left arm.

Things to Think About:

- You'll feel your biceps working as you lift, but especially at the midpoint of the movement.
- Avoid hunching over; keep your back naturally flat.
- Don't use any other part of your body to rock or force the weight upward.

Variations:

- **EASIER:** Do this exercise from a standing position; lean forward and allow your arm to hang down in front of you. Place your nonworking hand on a bench or your thigh for support.
- **HARDER:** Do this exercise while resting the back of your upper arm on a slanted bench called a preacher curl or Scott curl.

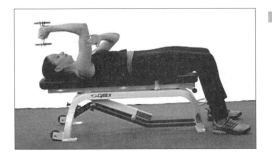

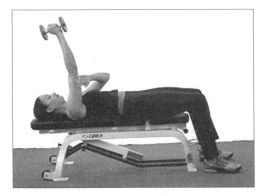

■ LYING KICK-OUTS

Muscles Worked: An excellent triceps isolator.

Joint Cautions: Slight elbow and shoulder caution.

Starting Position: Holding a dumbbell in your right hand, lie on a bench with your feet flat on the floor, hip width apart, or up on the bench if that's more comfortable. Extend your right arm straight up over your shoulder with your palm facing inward. Rest your left arm at your side or place it behind your right upper arm for support.

Exercise: Carefully bend your elbow and lower the weight until your thumb is level with your temple. Straighten your arm back up to the starting postion. Complete all reps and repeat with your left arm.

Things to Think About:
- Imagine you are trying to hammer something into the ceiling above you. You'll feel the muscles in the back of your upper arm working as you straighten your arm.
- Keep your shoulder stationary, using only your elbow to move the weight.

Variations:
- **EASIER:** Try the Kick Beats described on page 127.
- **HARDER:** Do this exercise with both arms at once.

WRIST CURLS

Muscles Worked: All of the muscles in your forearm are worked during this exercise.

Joint Cautions: None.

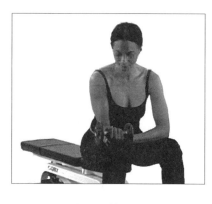

Starting Position: Hold a weight in your right hand with an underhand grip and sit on the edge of your bench with your feet hip width apart. Lean forward a little and place your entire forearm on top of your thigh so that your hand hangs over the edge of your knee. Place your left palm over your wrist.

Exercise: Curl your wrist up so that the dumbbell moves toward your forearm, and then lower the weight back down past the starting postion before moving into the next rep. Complete all reps and then repeat with the left wrist.

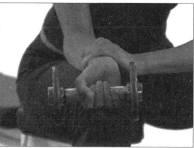

Things to Think About:
- This is a small, controlled movement. You'll feel the back and front of your forearms working as

you curl the weight upward. The tension will slowly build toward the end of the set.

- Don't overcurl; just lift until you feel the muscles working and then slowly lower.
- Don't hunch over; keep your back naturally flat.

Variations:

- **EASIER:** Do this exercise while standing and with your arms in front of your waist, your palms facing forward.
- **HARDER:** Roll the weight down the length of your fingers before curling back up to the starting position.

Advanced Upper-Body Training

To intensify upper-body training, try a technique known as super sets. This is when you do a set of one exercise and then immediately follow it—take absolutely zero rest between sets—with a different exercise, either for the same muscle group or for the muscle that performs the opposite function. Pairing a Lateral Raise and a Back Delt Fly is an intense and effective super set that targets the chest; doing a set of Concentration Curls immediately followed by a Lying Kick-out is a great oppositional super set that works the biceps and triceps.

Breakdown sets are another way to intensify your upper-body workout. To do a breakdown set, you start with the heaviest weight you can handle for, say, six to eight reps. When you tire out, you immediately pick up the next heaviest weight and do six to eight reps; repeat until you're using an extremely light weight. The idea here is to completely exhaust the muscle. Breakdowns work best with exercises such as Chest Flys, Back Delt Flys, and Lateral Raises where you work both sides of your body at the same time.

Both super sets and breakdown sets are for the intermediate or advanced exerciser.

The Arms Race

Women have 50–60 percent less upper-body strength than men, but only partly because of higher body fat percentage and a smaller capacity for building muscle mass in the top half of the body. Being "the weaker sex" is due mostly to the fact that women aren't typically the ones rearranging the furniture or operating heavy machinery, so they don't have much opportunity to beef up. When women do pump iron, the strength gap shrinks. If you think otherwise, check out these fantastic feats of female strength. You don't have to aspire to them, but they can inspire you nonetheless.

- The women's world record for discus throwing, 76.80 meters, is greater than the men's world record of 74.08 meters. (A men's discus is a few pounds heavier, but still . . .)

- The women's world record for chopping through a white pine log nine inches in diameter is 22.53 seconds. (The aptly named Shannon Strong set the record in 1998.)

- The longest distance a Frisbee has ever been thrown by a woman is 112 feet, 18 inches.

- The Women's United States Power Lifting Federation record for one repetition of a bench press is 352 pounds.

- In the World's Strongest Woman competition, contestants must, among other amazing demonstrations of raw power, pull a 10,000-pound truck more than sixty feet in ninety seconds and place a series of stones ranging from 70 to 150 pounds on top of a high wall.

8

THE PERFECT
STRENGTH WORKOUT

Amazingly, Jane was a two-pack-a-day smoker, grossly out of shape, and overweight until she was almost thirty. On her twenty-ninth birthday she woke up and decided to change her life by doing Jane Fonda videos in her apartment. When her neighbors complained, she joined a gym, and when she lost her job, she began a new career as a personal trainer and aerobics instructor. Somewhere along the line she quit smoking and began competing in National Aerobics Championship competitions, where she recently finished second in the masters' division. Now this forty-three-year-old keeps her body looking fit and strong with regular weight training, training for aerobic competitions, and boxing. "I love looking lean but muscular," she says. "And being strong makes me feel like I'm in control of my body as well as other aspects of my life."

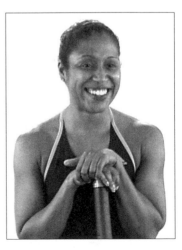

EXERCISES IN THIS CHAPTER
- Bench Presses
- Chin-ups
- Bar Rows
- Military Presses

- Bar Curls
- French Presses
- Power Squats
- Seated Calf Raises
- Bench V-Crunches
- Side Bridges

EQUIPMENT NEEDED

- A barbell
- Several sets of weight plates and weight collars or clips
- A weight bench
- A chin-up bar or chin-up frame

ESTIMATED WORKOUT TIME

- Beginners: 15–20 minutes, two or three times a week
- Intermediates: 15–20 minutes, four times a week (if you do a split routine) or 25–35 minutes, two or three times a week
- Advanced: 40 minutes, four times a week

Most people want to get stronger so they have more "real world" strength. They want to be able to conquer the real world of heavy doors, stubborn jars, and large pieces of furniture.

Scientifically speaking, real-world strength is not the true definition of strength. Strength as defined by exercise science nerds is the amount of force you can muster for one maximal effort, like an Olympic weight lifter hoisting a loaded barbell over his head or pushing out one repetition using maximum poundage on a bench press. When anyone else talks about strength, we're referring to muscular endurance. That's a fancy term for the amount of less-than-maximal force you can exert over some extended period of time. In other words, real-world strength.

Regardless of precise definitions, the idea of having physical strength is a relatively foreign concept for the average woman. Sure, it's nice to be able to rip open those sticky jars and push heavy things around the room, but is that enough of an impetus to get you into the weight room? Maybe not, but there are many other reasons why it's important to be strong, especially if you're a woman. Let me briefly mention a few:

- **It strengthens your bones.** When you think osteoporosis, you probably think of hunchbacked little old ladies with bones as delicate and breakable as eggshells. That's what my friend Hanna, a director of medical benefits for a large corporation, thought. Hanna has been a serious athlete her whole life. She runs, hikes, swims, and cycles; a few years ago she participated in an event called a Double Iron Man that requires participants to swim more than 5 miles, bike 240 miles, and run more than 50 miles—all on the same day! Since it's an established fact that weight-bearing exercise (activities such as walking and running, where you need to support your body weight during movement) does a good job of strengthening your bones, she assumed her bones were hard as diamonds.

  "While training for the double I had a total-body DEXA scan for bone density. I expected my bone density to be exceptional," she remembers. "I was more than unpleasantly surprised to learn that my bone density was average for a thirty-seven-year-old female."

  The fact is, there are ten million Americans who have osteoporosis—80 percent of them women—and some of them are as young as thirty. The National Osteoporosis Foundation expects this number to soar to forty-one million in the next ten years.

  As a medical expert and someone who takes her health seriously, Hanna began to read up on how to preserve her bone density. She soon found out that weight-bearing activity alone isn't enough to prevent bone deterioration. She realized that she—like all other women—would have to make a lifelong commitment to strength training.

  Strength training is an important part of preventing brittle bones, and some preliminary studies suggest that it may even reverse the condition to some extent. This is because strength training works your bones as well as your muscles. As your muscles move through strength exercises, they tug on your bones, stimulating them to create and store more calcium.

  Not only that, osteoporosis is joint-specific. It's possible to have dense bones in, say, your legs but have brittle bones in your upper body. The beauty of strengthening every area of your body is that you will stimulate all of your muscles and bones, not just a few select areas.

- **It reshapes your body.** Watching what you eat and doing regular cardio workouts will help you lose weight but don't have the power to change the shape and tone of a specific area on your body. Only strength training can do that.

   Strength training has the ability to spot-train. As most of my clients and regular readers know, "You cannot spot-reduce" has been one of my mantras for years. And it's true: There is no way to selectively zap fat off an area by exercising it. But strength training can tone, tighten, and firm the underlying muscles to change your appearance.

   Does that mean you can turn yourself into a long, lithe dancer if your basic frame is short and compact? Of course not. But you can enhance the bone structure you were born with. You can make your hips appear smaller by strengthening and reshaping your shoulders to even out your proportions. You can make your breasts look younger and perkier by bolstering the pectoral muscles that reside beneath them. You can strengthen your abdominals so you stand up straighter and look leaner.

   Plus, I happen to think strong-looking women are sexy. Terri Walsh, a personal trainer and fitness model who is well known in New York for her killer body, is a perfect example. Though she's very feminine, she looks like she can clean-and-jerk a bus over her head. "Being a jock chick doesn't mean you have to look like a guy," she says. "I am really reaping the benefits of strength training as I get older—no one believes that I'm thirty-eight years old."

- **It helps you lose weight.** Yup. You read that right. If you're serious about losing weight, then you'd better be serious about strength training. (My clients and regular readers will recognize this as another one of my favorite mantras.)

   The reason strength training is so effective for promoting weight loss is that it builds muscle, which burns more calories than fat. Stacks of research tell us that for every additional pound of muscle you pack onto your body, you burn an additional 30 to 50 calories daily. I know that doesn't sound like a lot, but it's actually pretty significant. Even this tiny uptick in your metabolism can have a potentially big payoff; it can translate into a weight loss (or prevention of weight gain) of three to five pounds of fat a year. That's the power of adding just one additional pound of muscle; do the math on what adding several pounds of muscle can do for you.

By the way, some of this fat loss may not necessarily show up as a loss of scale weight because muscle is denser than fat. One pound of muscle takes up about 20 percent less room than a pound of fat.

- **It augments your health.** It's obvious that stronger muscles, joints, and bones add up to fewer injuries, but weight training offers other significant health benefits as well. For instance, did you know that it helps prevent heart disease and may help you recover more quickly from a heart attack? A recent study done at the Carolinas Medical Center in Charlotte—among many other studies—found that subjects who strength-trained recovered more quickly from a heart episode than those who did cardio alone or nothing at all, because strength training increases lean body mass, decreases body fat, and eases stresses on the body. Some preliminary studies suggest that strength training may also help in the prevention and treatment of cancer, including breast cancer.

- **It strengthens your self-esteem.** Plus One Fitness, the fitness management company I work for, recently introduced our Athena Women's Strength Training program into our corporate fitness centers. Named after the Greek goddess of wisdom, these eight-week, women-only sessions include hands-on instructions on how to use free weights and how to structure a free-weight training program. We introduced this program in response to the fact that our weight-training areas were packed—but not with women.

Although women's participation in strength training has nearly tripled, from 6.8 million to 18.6 million, in the last decade, most women have gravitated toward resistance machines and body-sculpting classes. While we didn't feel there was anything wrong with this trend, we believe women should have the skills, knowledge, and confidence to use free weights.

Athena has been a huge success for Plus One. Every eight-week session has been fully subscribed from the get-go. The women who go through the program get stronger and learn new skills. For instance, a recent Athena group began with none of the women capable of performing a military-style push-up, a chin-up, or a bench press of over 50 pounds. At the end of eight weeks, every single woman—many of them over forty years old—was able to do at least ten military-style push-ups with perfect form. The majority were able to do at least one pull-up. All could bench-press over 50 pounds, with one woman pressing a whopping 115 pounds.

None of this is surprising. But what is surprising—at least to me— is the strong personal and emotional response women have to Athena.

Having physical strength makes them feel empowered, better able to take on the world beyond the weight room. This is what Pam, a recent Athena graduate, has to say about the program: "Strength training is where I learn how to be strong physically and mentally. Each training session becomes a challenge that I meet with dedication, hard work, mental focus, physical power, and stamina. In my daily life strength training has improved my confidence and my determination to succeed." Her thoughts are mirrored by virtually every Athena graduate.

Now most of our free-weight rooms are about half men and half women.

The Rules for Building Strength

Building strength is part science, part art—part science because there are certain things that hold true no matter what, part art because it often requires a little experimentation and creativity to get the results you want. Remember, we're building real-world strength here, so the parameters I've laid out for you are aimed at this goal.

Training for strength involves understanding and controlling the variables, or components, of your workout. These components include the amount of weight you lift, the number of repetitions you do per set, the number of sets you do, the amount of rest you take, proper technique, and the type of exercise you choose. Let's discuss each of these variables in detail.

- **Amount of weight.** Getting stronger means lifting heavy weights. I hope that's not a shocking statement. If you have a fear of lifting heavy weights because you're concerned about bulking up, you need to get over it. Most women, no matter how much weight they lift, do not pile on mountains of muscle. Unless you spend hours and hours in the gym and have an unusual amount of male hormones coursing through your bloodstream, it's not likely you'll blow up like some sort of giant muscle balloon. You'll have to trust me on this one.

  Now that we've put this fear to bed, you should be comfortable lifting a heavy enough weight so that you have to push yourself to complete the last few repetitions of every set. While you should still be able to maintain good form throughout, those last few reps should challenge every fiber of the muscle you're targeting.

- **Repetitions.** Training for strength means doing fewer repetitions per set than training for shape or tone. Typically, you'll aim for six to eight reps per set. Since you're lifting the weight fewer times, you can handle heavier poundage. Once you can lift a weight eight times with good technique, you should increase the weight and drop down to the lower end of the repetition range.

- **Sets.** No matter what type of goals you're pointed toward, beginners should always start out by doing one set per exercise for several workouts. This is especially true when you're training for strength: Since you're lifting heavy weights and doing exercises that involve a great deal of muscle usage, the potential for injury and extreme soreness is high.

  After the first few weeks of training, however, you should up your workload to three to five sets per exercise. For multiple sets I recommend using the "sandwich" approach: your first set is a warm-up to introduce the muscles to the exercise, the middle sets are the "meat" of the workout, where you really give it your all; and the final set is the cool-down or transition to the next exercise. This means you'll lift a somewhat lighter weight for your first set of an exercise, bump it up to a heavier weight for the one to three sets in the middle, and take it down for the last set.

There are other advanced techniques and approaches to multiple set training (as I discuss in the "Advanced Weight-Training Techniques" sidebar on page 173), but the sandwich approach serves as a good foundation for strength training.

- **Rest.** There are two types of rest involved in strength training: the rest you take between sets, and the rest you take between workouts.

  Strength building requires more rest between sets than other types of weight training because you want to give your muscles adequate time to recover so they're ready to go for the next big effort. I recommend you take as much time as you feel you need between sets. This can mean as little as ninety seconds and as much as three minutes. More rest slows your workout down, but it will deliver better results.

  Rest between workouts can be somewhat more complicated. Generally, muscles perform best if they have at least forty-eight hours off between workouts, especially heavy workouts. So you have a choice. You can work your entire body all in one shot, or you can split up your routine over the course of several days. Since strength training takes a little longer, I find that many exercisers opt for the split.

  The best way to split up your workout? You have a couple of options. You can work your upper body one day and your lower body the next, or you can pair muscles that work in tandem with each other on the same day, such as the "pull" muscles of your back and biceps and the "push" muscles of your chest and triceps.

  The split you choose is a matter of personal preference and how your body responds. You may have to experiment to find your optimal routine. My body always seems to respond better to an upper-body/lower-body split. I feel like I can devote all of my energy to the muscles I'm working without having to worry about tiring out support and oppositional muscles. I usually (but not always) work my middle muscles with my lower body. But again, this is my personal preference. The other way isn't wrong. I've outlined both options in the exercise section.

- **Technique.** To maximize strength, good technique is essential. Heck, it's always essential. With strength workouts, technique can get you better results. Let me give you an example. Say you do a bench press to work your chest but you always arch your back. This displaces a lot of energy to your lower back muscles, energy you could be devoting to strengthening your chest muscles. If you also quickly bounce the bar off your chest rather than moving slowly through the exercise, you don't give a large percentage of your muscle fibers a chance to catch up with the movement and get into the act. You may be able to lift more weight using momentum, but you certainly won't develop much strength.

- **Choice of exercises.** Almost any exercise you perform correctly will help you develop strength. But I think some exercises are better suited to true strength training than others. I chose the exercises in this chapter because they work groups of muscles in teams rather than in isolation. This is the way you use your muscles in everyday life, so it stands to reason that this is the most efficient way to develop real-world strength. There are other exercises that fit the bill, but I've attempted to select the classics, the exercises that are the most basic and the most tried-and-true in traditional strength training. They're among the top choices of professional athletes and dedicated weight lifters.

The Perfect Strength Exercises

All levels of exercisers should warm up thoroughly before a strength-training workout. Five to ten minutes of easy cycling, brisk walking, or Active-Isolated stretching (see chapter 10) will get your blood flowing and heat up your muscles so they can move more fluidly. Don't skip the warm-up to save time—it's essential for injury prevention. Research also shows that you're more likely to have a productive workout if you warm up properly.

Your cool-down should mirror your warm-up, but I also recommend adding some stretching to counterbalance your weight work. The Perfect Stretch Workout or the Perfect Mind-Body Workout are both excellent cool-down choices.

I'm often asked if it's okay to do a full-blown cardio workout on the same day as a weight workout. My answer depends on what your ultimate goals are. If building strength is your absolute priority, then you may want to alternate your cardio and strength training days, or at the very least save your cardio until after you've hit the weights. But if you also consider weight loss a primary goal, then I recommend doing at least some cardio every day.

Beginners should start with one set of each exercise listed in this chapter, six to ten repetitions per set. Do the entire workout in one session, taking at least ninety seconds of rest between sets. Use a weight that is challenging yet doable—by the last rep you should still be able to maintain impeccable form but your muscles should feel completely worked.

Ideally, you want to perform this workout three times per week, with at least one day off in between workouts. (It's okay to continue your cardio workouts in between.) If you find you are so sore that picking up a fork or walking to the mailbox is an excruciating event even several days after your workout, you've overdone it. In this case you'll need to back off on workout intensity, which usually means lightening up on the weights and increasing the amount of reps per set. You may also want to try the easier variation listed for each exercise.

Once you begin to flow through the entire routine comfortably, without feeling too sore or tired afterward, up your workload to two sets per exercise. When you can blow through this routine with no problem, consider yourself an intermediate.

Intermediates will do two to four sets of each of the exercises listed in this chapter, six to eight reps per set. Your weights should remain challenging and you should continue to rest as much as you need to in between sets.

Although each of the exercises in this chapter works several muscle groups at once, they all depend on a "prime mover" muscle to take the lead and do the bulk of the work. Prime movers include the buttocks, quadriceps, hamstrings, calves, upper back, chest, shoulders, triceps, biceps, and abdominals and lower back. Ideally, you want to exercise each prime mover at least twice a week. If you have time, you can perform the entire routine in one session. If you don't, I recommend choosing one of the following split-routine options. Alternate training days so that you do each workout twice in one week.

- **Option 1** (upper-body/lower-body split)
  - Day 1: Bench Presses, Chin-ups, Bar Rows, Military Presses, Bar Curls, French Presses
  - Day 2: Power Squats, Seated Calf Raises, Bench V-Crunches, Side Bridges
- **Option 2** (push [lower-body]/pull [middle-body] split)
  - Day 1: Bench Presses, Power Squats, Military Presses, Seated Calf Raises, French Presses
  - Day 2: Chin-ups, Bench V-Crunches, Bar Rows, Side Bridges, Bar Curls

When you feel your workouts are under control and you're ready to push yourself a little harder, move on to the advanced routine.

Advanced exercisers should perform three to five sets of each of the exercises listed in this chapter, six to eight repetitions per set. Rest between sets and workouts should remain the same. You have the option of doing your entire routine in one day or splitting it up as described in the intermediate section. You'll probably get better strength results by splitting up your routine. Advanced exercisers should do at least some of their sets using the harder variation listed for each exercise.

During the first few weeks of weight training you may see some strength gains. These early improvements have more to do with improvements in technique and how your brain processes the impulses from your muscles.

The real strength gains come after about six weeks of training, when improvements in strength have more to do with muscular development. Don't be surprised if you make a huge leap in the amount of work you're able to do at about the six-week mark.

Besides getting stronger, you'll also see other changes in your body after about six to eight weeks: Your muscles will be firmer and more shapely, and if you've kept up with your cardio workouts and watched your diet, you'll look leaner and smaller even if there's no corresponding drop in scale weight.

■ BENCH PRESSES

Muscles Worked: This is the ultimate chest-strengthening exercise. It also works the shoulders and triceps.

Joint Cautions: Shoulder, rotator cuff, neck, and lower back.

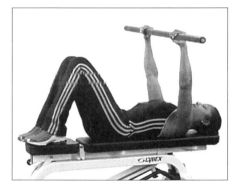

Starting Position: Lie on the bench with your feet flat on the floor or up on the bench if that is more comfortable. Grip the bar so that your arms are evenly spaced and a few inches wider than shoulder width apart. Lie naturally without forcing your back into the pad. Lift the bar off the stanchions (the rack system that it rests on) and straighten your arms upward so that your elbows remain slightly bent and they are directly over your shoulders.

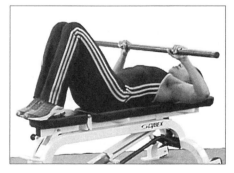

Exercise: Lower the bar until your elbows are slightly below your shoulders and then press back up to the starting position.

Things to Think About:
- Experts used to tell people to lower the bar until it bounced off the chest, but this is

extremely hard on the shoulders and rotator cuff. Lowering until the elbows are slightly below the shoulders is not only safer but a more effective way to strengthen the chest muscles.

- Avoid arching your back as you press the weight upward. If you feel you need to arch your back, chances are the weight is too heavy.

Variations:

- EASIER: If you find this exercise is too rough on your shoulders, try the Incline Dumbbell Presses, described on page 140.
- HARDER: Move your hands a few inches closer together. This will factor out some of the assistance your chest receives from your triceps.

■ CHIN-UPS

Muscles Worked: Chin-ups target the back, shoulders, and biceps.

Joint Cautions: Shoulders, rotator cuff, elbows.

Starting Position: Stand in front of a pull-up bar and jump up to grab the bar with your hands a few inches apart and your palms facing toward you. Keep your body naturally straight with your legs together.

Exercise: Bend your arms to lift your body upward. When your arms are fully bent and your upper chest is above the level of the bar, slowly lower yourself to the starting position. Complete all of your reps before you carefully let go of the bar and return to the floor.

Things to Think About:

- You'll feel a strong pull through your upper arms and the wings of your back as you pull upward.
- Be careful not to overarch your back or rock your body to lift yourself upward.
- Keep your shoulders down and relaxed.

Variations:

- EASIER: Bend your knees and cross one ankle over the other; you can have a spotter assist you by holding on to your feet. Many gyms also have assisted pull-up/chin-up machines that partially counterbalance

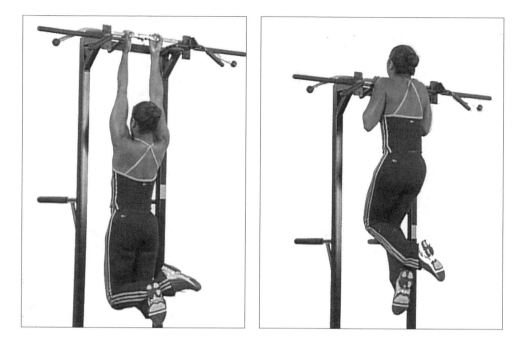

your weight. This is an ideal variation if you aren't strong enough to perform this exercise.

- **HARDER:** Place your hands shoulder width apart and turn your palms forward. *Note:* Avoid behind-the-neck pull-ups. They are very hard on your shoulders and rotator cuff.

▪ BAR ROWS

Muscles Worked: Besides the upper and middle back, this exercise also strengthens the shoulders and biceps.

Joint Cautions: Lower back.

Starting Position: Place a bar on the floor or on top of a low platform and stand in front of it with your feet hip width apart. Pull your abs in, bend your knees a few inches, and lean forward from the hips to grasp the bar with your hands about shoulder width apart and your palms facing downward. Lift the bar off the floor so that your arms

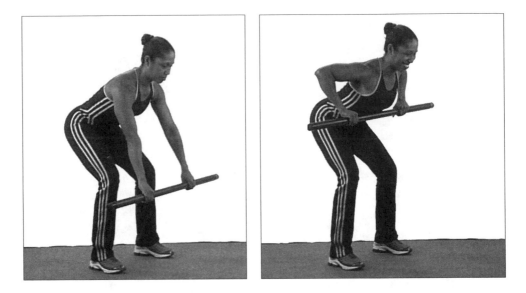

are hanging straight downward and your torso is at a 45-degree angle with the floor.

Exercise: While maintaining your body positioning, bend your arms to move the bar toward your chest. When the bar is a few inches in front of your chest, slowly lower to the starting postion.

Things to Think About:
- Imagine you are trying to start a large lawn mower by pulling the start cord toward you.
- Keeping your body stable and in the proper position protects your lower back and ensures that only the muscles you're supposed to be using get a workout.
- Avoid arching your back or rounding it.
- Avoid jerking the bar upward or letting the bar down too quickly to the start. This can be hard on your lower back, shoulders, and elbows.

Variations:
- **EASIER:** Turn your palms upward so that the biceps are in a stronger position to assist the movement.
- **HARDER:** Do this exercise extra slowly.

■ MILITARY PRESSES

Muscles Worked: The all-time great shoulder-strengthening exercise. Works your upper back and arms, too.

Joint Cautions: Shoulders, rotator cuff, neck.

Starting Position: Sit up tall on a weight bench. You can either lean back and use the backrest for support or, if you feel more comfortable and have a strong lower back, sit up tall without using back support. With your elbows bent, place your hands (palms forward) on the bar a few inches wider than shoulder width apart. Sit tall with your abs pulled inward and your back comfortably against the seat. Lift the bar off the stanchions so that your hands are level with your collarbone.

Exercise: Press the bar upward by straightening your arms. Lower slowly until your elbows are slightly below shoulder level and then press back upward. When you have completed the last rep, lower all the way back to the start, then place the bar carefully back on the stanchions.

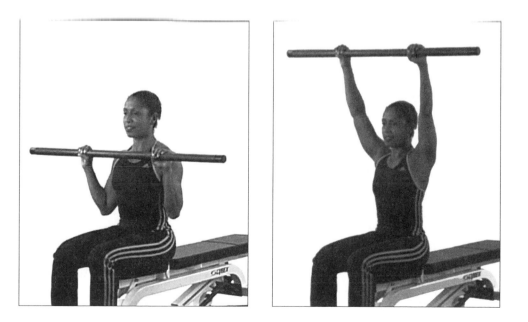

Things to Think About:

- Never modify this exercise so that you bring the bar behind your neck. This is one of the single most damaging moves for your rotator cuff and shoulders.
- Take care not to arch your back off the seat as you lift the bar.
- Focus on lowering only until your elbows are slightly below your shoulders; leave some bend in your elbows as you press back up to the start.

Variations:

- EASIER: Have a spotter help you guide the bar through this exercise, and use back support.
- HARDER: Use a military chair without a back support, but do this version only if you are completely comfortable with this exercise and you have no lower back issues.

■ BAR CURLS

Muscles Worked: A great isolation exercise to strengthen the biceps.

Joint Cautions: Mild caution for lower back, elbows.

Starting Position: While standing tall with your feet hip width apart, hold a bar in both hands with your palms facing upward and your hands slightly wider than shoulder width apart. Bend your knees slightly and pull your abs inward.

Exercise: Bend your elbows to curl the bar up to your shoulders and then slowly straighten your arms back to the starting position.

Things to Think About:

- When you do this exercise correctly, you'll feel a strong pull through the center front of your arms, especially as you are bending your arms upward and they move through the point where they're parallel to the floor.
- Avoid arching backward as you lift the bar or leaning forward to lower the bar.

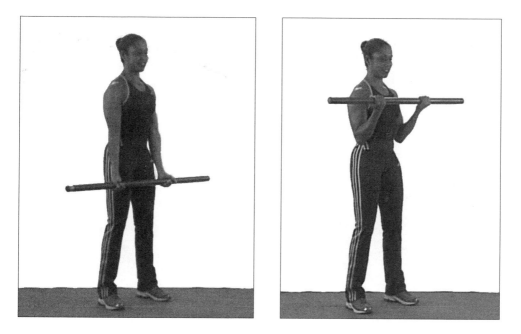

- Move slowly and with control to avoid snapping your shoulders or elbows.

Variations:

- **EASIER:** Try the Concentration Curls as described on page 145.
- **HARDER:** Do a bar curl from a preacher bench; this is a seated bench with a pad that you rest your elbows on so that your arms hang down at an angle.

FRENCH PRESSES

Muscles Worked: A great move for strengthening your triceps.

Joint Cautions: Mild caution for shoulders, elbows, wrists.

Starting Position: Hold on to a straight or bent bar with your palms facing forward and lie on a bench with your feet down on the floor or, if you're short, up on the bench. Contract your abs. Lift the bar straight up over your shoulders.

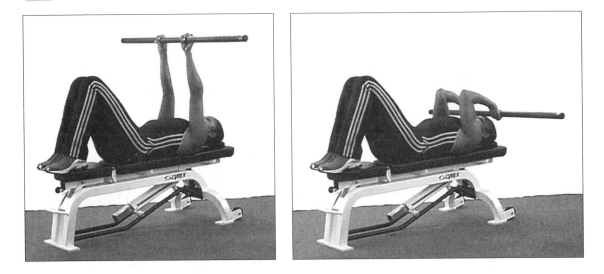

Exercise: Slowly bend your arms to lower the bar toward your forehead. When it is an inch or so above your forehead, straighten your arms back up.

Things to Think About:
- Think of your arms as a door and your elbows as a hinge. Your arms should remain in alignment as your elbows move.
- You'll feel a strong pull through the back of your upper arms as you press the bar upward.
- Keep your shoulders relaxed, down, and still. Keep your wrists in line with the rest of your arm. Avoid completely locking your elbows at the top of the movement.

Variations:
- **EASIER:** If this exercise bothers your elbows, try a Lying Kick-out as described on page 146.
- **HARDER:** Have a spotter lightly press inward on the outside of your elbows. This will help isolate the triceps.

■ POWER SQUATS

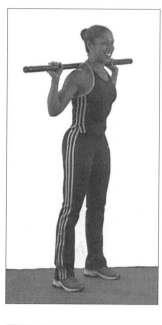

Muscles Worked: A true workhorse of an exercise. Besides strengthening the buttocks and thighs, this exercise works virtually every muscle in your body in one way or another.

Joint Cautions: Lower back, knees.

Starting Position: Place a bar across the back of your shoulders and place your hands on the bar a comfortable distance apart. (You can place a pad or towel across your neck if the bar puts too much pressure on you.) Stand tall with your feet hip width apart and your abs contracted.

Exercise: Bend your knees until you find your upper body folding forward or until your thighs are parallel to the floor. How far down you can go depends on your flexibility. Once you reach the bottom of the movement, hold a moment and then, exercising control, "explode" back up to the starting postion by straightening your knees.

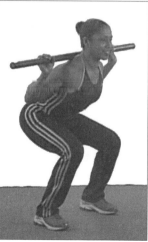

Things to Think About:
* As you sit backward and downward, imagine you're sitting down into a chair that's been placed directly behind you. You'll feel a strong pull through your thighs and, possibly, your buttocks as you both lift and lower.
* Avoid allowing yourself to fold too far forward or allowing your knees to move forward of your toes.
* Never lower yourself so that your thighs are below parallel to the floor.

Variations:
* **EASIER:** Do the basic version of the Half Squat as described on page 54. You can also perform this exercise in a Smith machine, a large frame that has guide rods for the bar.
* **HARDER:** Hold the bar across the top of your chest. Cross your arms and hold on to the bar.

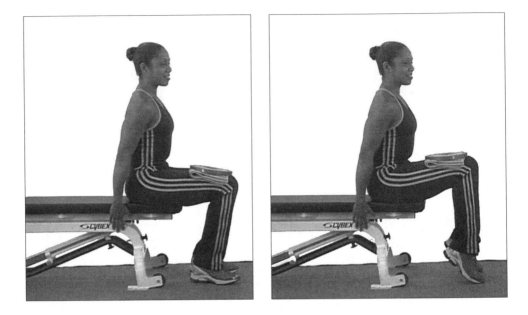

■ SEATED CALF RAISES

Muscles Worked: Most calf exercises work the muscles closest to the surface. This exercise also targets the deeper muscles of the calf.

Joint Cautions: Mild caution for ankles.

Starting Position: Sit up tall in a chair with your feet hip width apart. Place a weight plate across your thighs, just above your knees. (You can place a pad or a towel in between.) Place your hands on the plate to balance it, or place them on the sides of the bench.

Exercise: Lift your heels up off the floor as high as you can. Hold a moment and then lower your heels back to the start.

Things to Think About:
- You'll feel a strong contraction through the center of your calves, especially at the top of the movement.
- Keep your ankles straight as you lift and lower your heels.

Variations:

- **EASIER:** Rather than placing a plate on your thighs, simply use your hands to apply resistance as you raise your heels. Some gyms have seated calf machines that mimic this exercise.
- **HARDER:** Place your feet on a low platform so that your heels are hanging off. Lower your heels past the starting position.

■ BENCH V-CRUNCHES

Muscles Worked: A killer strengthening exercise for your abs and lower back.

Joint Cautions: Strong caution for the lower back.

Starting Position: Sit up tall on the edge of the bench with your abs pulled inward and your hands gripping either side of the bench. Bend your elbows and lean back so your feet come off the floor and are level with the top of the bench.

Exercise: Fold your upper and lower body together by simultaneously bending your knees in toward your chest and straightening your arms to bring your upper body forward to meet your knees. Hold a moment and stretch back out to the starting position.

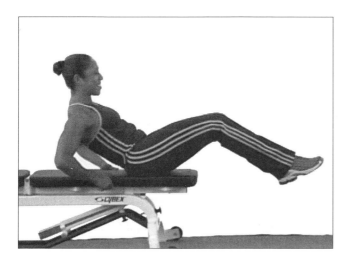 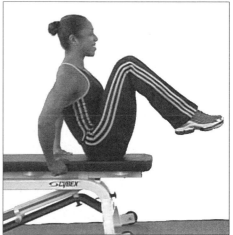

Things to Think About:

• Think of your body as an accordion, moving smoothly together and apart. You'll feel your abs contracting very strongly at the top of the movement and as you stretch back out to the starting position.

• Focus on keeping your abs strongly contracted and your spine straight to protect your lower back.

Variations:

• EASIER: Hold your legs below the bench and don't fold your upper and lower body as closely together.

• HARDER: Hold a light dumbbell between your feet.

■ SIDE BRIDGES

Muscles Worked: Although all of your abdominal muscles work during this exercise, it places special emphasis on your internal and external obliques.

Joint Cautions: Lower back, neck.

Starting Position: Lie on your left side with your legs out straight, stacked directly one on top of the other, and slightly forward of your hips. Place your right hand behind your head and place your left elbow and forearm on the floor.

Exercise: Pull your abs inward and engage them to lift your torso and hips off the floor. Hold a moment at the top of the movement and slowly return to the starting position. Do an equal number of reps with both your right and left sides.

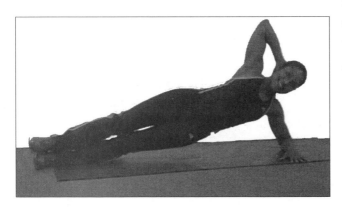

Things to Think About:

• You'll feel a strong pull through your waist as you lift upward.

• Make sure your hips are stacked directly on top of each other to ensure proper alignment for your lower back.

- Keep your entire body in a straight line as you stay lifted; don't arch your lower back or hunch your shoulders.

Variations:
- EASIER: Use your right hand to steady and balance the movement rather than placing your hand behind your head.
- HARDER: As you hold the up position, lift your top leg up a few inches.

Advanced Weight-Training Techniques

One way to jump-start your weight-training routine is by trying out new training methods. Doing a standard move a different way often makes it feel like a completely new exercise. Three new tricks to try:

- **Pyramids.** If you are focusing on a particular exercise or your goal is to lift a specific amount of weight, consider using pyramid sets, that is, doing four or five sets of the same exercise starting with light weight and high reps (eight to fifteen) and gradually working your way up to the heaviest weight you can lift for one or two repetitions. The bench press is a classic pyramid exercise because your one-rep max (the heaviest weight you can lift one time) is subject to bragging rights.

- **Reverse pyramids.** You can also do reverse pyramid sets by starting with the heaviest weights and fewest reps and gradually working lighter with each succeeding set. Though not a technique recommended for beginners, it's an effective way for more-experienced lifters to hoist their heaviest possible poundage.

- **Negatives.** Forget the old standard "accentuate the positive, eliminate the negative." In weight training, the negative phase—when you lower the weight—is just as important for building strength as the positive or lifting phase. Negative training involves getting some assistance with the lift from a spotter or partner and then slowly, slowly lowering the weight to make the most of the negative. This is a great technique for anyone who's having trouble graduating to the next weight up on the rack or who wants to push through a plateau.

Strong Opinions

When *Newsweek* did a cover story on a weight-training technique called SuperSlow a few years ago, I was swamped with questions—even my mom wanted to know if it was something she should be doing.

The SuperSlow technique is weight training at a snail's pace; you take about sixty seconds to complete each repetition. Proponents say it's effective because it works your muscles more deeply and thoroughly. It's safer because you move too slowly to strain anything.

My opinion? SuperSlow can build a decent amount of strength and muscle size, and if you're looking for a time-efficient workout, it's an option to consider. However, the SuperSlow method loses all credibility for some of the other theories associated with it. For instance, believers eschew other forms of exercise, especially cardiovascular, dismissing them as dangerous and ineffective.

When asked to back up such outrageous claims, Ken Hutchins, president of the SuperSlow Guild, offers this neatly bundled argument: The mountain of evidence showing the positive effects of other types of exercise is null and void because *all* exercise research uses flawed methods, reports incorrect data, and is performed by incompetent investigators. (By the way, this isn't just hearsay; I've had an ongoing personal dialogue with Hutchins for several years now.)

As any exercise professional worth his or her salt will tell you, there is overwhelming proof of the positive effects offered by cardiovascular exercise and many other workouts. And exercise scientists use the same time-honored methods used by other established areas of research, including technology, math, physics, and chemistry.

I won't tell you to stay away from SuperSlow because I believe it can be a valid way to strength-train. It's a shame that SuperSlow advocates have taken a kernel of truth and mucked it up with pseudoscience and flat-out lies for the sake of getting sound bites in the media. I caution you to approach SuperSlow with eyes—and brain—wide open.

Sizable Matters

Even though the majority of women don't possess enough of the male hormone, testosterone, to build gargantuan muscles no matter how much iron they pump, many women shy away from weight training for fear of bulking up. Some of them turn to alternatives such as Pilates and yoga, which advertise their ability to build strength without bulk. But do these activities offer much in the way of strength benefits? And if so, do they really prevent your muscles from gaining size?

"Pilates and yoga do build strength (to a degree) without bulk," comments Richard Cotton, M.A., vice president and chief exercise physiologist for First Fitness, Inc., in Utah. According to Cotton, both workouts feature low resistance and a higher number of repetitions of an exercise compared to a strength-building routine. "Beginning exercisers will build strength with yoga and Pilates but they will eventually plateau unless they add more resistance. They will never get to the absolute strength of a weight trainer," he adds.

9

THE PERFECT GYM WORKOUT

On the day Courtney turned twenty-five, she broke up with her boyfriend, signed up for college courses, gave up smoking, and started working out. She admits it was hard to get started, but once she got into a regular fitness routine that consists primarily of weight training, walking on the treadmill, and using the stair-climbing machine, she saw results fairly quickly. "One day after a few months of working out I was blow-drying my hair and noticed my arms had definition," she remembers with a laugh. "That's when I really knew I was on to something." Courtney almost always works out in a gym because she draws energy and motivation from having other people around. She also likes the variety of equipment a gym offers. "I'm not limited to just the equipment I have at home, so I can change my routine whenever I feel like it," she says.

EXERCISES IN THIS CHAPTER

- Leg Presses
- Leg Curls
- Inner Thigh Machine
- Machine Calf Raises
- Lat Pull-downs
- Chest Presses

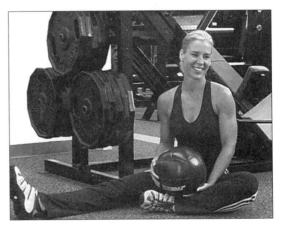

- Shoulder Press Machine
- Cable Biceps Curls
- Cable Triceps Extensions
- Hanging Knee-ups

EQUIPMENT NEEDED

- Leg press machine
- Leg curl machine
- Outer/inner thigh machine
- Lat pull-down machine
- Chest press machine
- Shoulder press machine
- Cable machine
- Ab straps or a captain's chair

ESTIMATED WORKOUT TIME

- Beginner: 15–20 minutes two to four times a week
- Intermediate: 25–35 minutes, two to four times a week
- Advanced: 35–45 minutes, two to four times a week

I love gyms! I love them so much, I've made a career out of designing and managing them. On the weekends I go visit other companies' gyms. When I travel I make it a point to see what's going on in gyms around the area I'm visiting. I love everything about gyms: the equipment, the classes, the people, the energy.

Others share my love of gyms. Bette, for example, started out as a client in one of my corporate gyms. She enjoyed working out there so much that she quit her job in the financial industry and came to work for us. "I felt confident that I could combine my business experience and passion for fitness to teach others about exercise and healthy living," she says. She's now a general manager at one of our more upscale hotel gyms—or fitness centers, as some of our tonier places are called. She says it has been the most rewarding career move of her life.

This chapter is for people like Bette, me, and the millions of others in this country who also love to work out in a gym and want to make the most of the experience. However, I should warn you that gyms are not for everyone.

Join the Club

As much as I love gyms and think they're great, not everyone is going to share this feeling. Some people value the privacy and flexibility of working out at home. I often find that beginning exercisers, especially if they need to lose a lot of weight, are too self-conscious to join a gym, let alone show up at one in workout clothes. Others don't like to be cooped up, or they seek the freedom and independence of the open road. Before you plunk down your cash, you should evaluate whether or not owning a gym membership is right for you. Here's a quick rundown of the type of person whose fitness routine will thrive in a gym.

- **People who want help with their workouts.** A gym is the most likely place to find seasoned fitness professionals who are certified, experienced, and knowledgeable. Having access to this type of assistance is invaluable. Working with a good trainer takes much of the guesswork out of your workout routine. It often makes the difference between success and failure. Read the "How to Choose a Trainer" sidebar on page 201 to evaluate whether or not a gym's staff is up to standard.

- **People who like to take group classes.** Most gyms have a variety of classes on their schedule, so you can sample a wide range of programs, from yoga and spinning to kickboxing and swing dance aerobics. The schedule usually changes every few months or so, so you're constantly exposed to new ideas and never get bored. In ideal circumstances, the instructors are certified, knowledgeable, and attentive, and the feedback you get from them is valuable for advancing your fitness routine.

- **People who like a lot of equipment.** Exercise equipment is in constant evolution. The elliptical trainer, one of the most popular pieces of cardio equipment, didn't even exist until about five years ago. Typically, the most interesting advances in exercise equipment take place within the gym. Gyms can afford the big bucks it takes to constantly update to the latest and greatest machines; they need to do this in order to stay competitive. Most of us don't have the cash flow to change our home exercise equipment once every six months or so, and even if we did, it isn't our job to keep up with minute-by-minute advances. New exercise machine ideas do eventually trickle down to home versions of machines, but they are often inferior imitations.

• **People who thrive on group energy.** What better place to find others who are like-minded about a healthy lifestyle than in a gym? It's a place to socialize and still get in a workout! You can almost always find a workout partner or, at the very least, people to encourage you. When my mom began her weight loss and shape-up effort, I signed her up at a local gym. At first she was a little intimidated to walk through the doors. She thought that she would be the only one who was not in perfect shape and assumed all of the hard bodies would be very judgmental of her. To the contrary. Everyone, staff and fellow members alike, was supportive, and many of them went out of their way to compliment her when her efforts obviously began to pay off. To her surprise, some of her biggest supporters turned out to be those hard bodies she had found so intimidating.

Weighing Your Options

In the above section I told you all about the wonderful things gyms have to offer. This may make you want to run out and join the first gym you see. Resist that urge. I was describing the ideal, the best of circumstances. There are more than twenty thousand gyms in the United States today, and trust me—they are *not* all created equal. While most strive to meet their members' needs, there are lemons.

And let me tell you, gym memberships do not always come cheap. In some parts of the country you can purchase a membership for around

$150 a year. Gyms memberships in large cities such as New York, Los Angeles, or Chicago can go for as high as $10,000 a year. That's a lot of green.

If you decide to join a gym, you owe it to yourself to dedicate a little thought and time to researching what's out there and deciding what will work best for you. You should treat the purchase of a gym membership just as you would any other important and costly decision, such as buying a car or a refrigerator. This means never purchasing a membership sight unseen. You'll need to visit every gym you consider joining and give it a thorough once-over. I recommend using the following checklist to help determine whether or not a gym is the right fit for you.

- **National chains versus local gyms.** There are a growing number of national gym chains that boast as many as a thousand centers tied together in one large network. This can be an advantage if you travel a lot or if you have a busy schedule. Town Sports International, for instance, has a New York Sports Club in just about every neighborhood in New York City as well as clubs in New Jersey, Connecticut, and Pennsylvania; commuters have the flexibility of working out near their home or workplace. When they travel to other parts of the country for business or pleasure, there are affiliated gyms in almost every major and not-so-major city. Bally's, Lifetime, Gold's, World Gym, and the YMCA are just a few examples of other national gym chains.

    Chains also have the advantage of critical mass. Their facilities are generally much larger than stand-alone gyms, so the locker rooms, group classrooms, exercise floor, and other areas are often more spacious. They get better prices on equipment, so they can afford more of it, more often. They attract top trainers and instructors because there is opportunity for professional growth. They usually have extensive group class schedules as well a large personal-training staff, spa, baby-sitting, and countless other amenities.

    So why would anyone join a stand-alone gym, a gym that only has one location? Because, like the TV show *Cheers*, when you go there everyone will know your name. Usually stand-alone gyms are smaller, neighborhood operations owned by a dedicated individual who is passionate about getting people into shape. You may sacrifice the oversized locker rooms and the eighty-class-a-week schedule, but you'll get coziness and personal attention in return. If there is a convenient, quality stand-alone fitness center near you and you don't travel much, it may be the better choice.

- **Location.** Studies show that if it takes you more than ten minutes to get to your gym, there is little chance you will use it on a regular basis. All other things being equal, the gym that is closer to you is the one you're most likely to use. Do some thinking about this. If you plan on working out in the morning, look for a gym near your house. If you have a job and plan on exercising in the evening, you may be better off joining something near work. Even if you decide to buy a membership in a chain, scout out their most convenient locations.

  The only exception to this rule is if you participate in a specialty workout such as rock climbing, sand volleyball, or boxing and the best (or only) facilities for your passion are located farther away. If you're dedicated to your sport or fitness activity, you're going to travel as far as it takes to participate. I myself travel to an out-of-the-way rock-climbing gym.

- **When you will work out.** It's a good idea to club-shop at the time of day you plan on working out. That's the only way to get a feel for what's happening at the time you'll be exercising. Most clubs are busiest on Monday nights. If you visit the club at that time and there is a thirty-minute wait for the cardio machines and the exercise floor is so crowded that people have to step sideways past each other, think twice about joining. Look for a location that's less packed during your workout time.

- **Staff.** Most clubs offer the same type of equipment, the same type of classes, and the same type of amenities. So what makes a club great?

  "Although I've worked at dozens and dozens of gyms, I've maintained my primary membership at the same one for nineteen years. Why? Because I like the staff and they help create an atmosphere conducive to working out," says John, a writer from Long Island who belongs to a small group of clubs called Eastern Athletic Clubs.

The time to find out about the staff is when you're club shopping. When you walk in, are they tightly clustered in groups gossiping about the members, or does someone come right up and greet you? Are there trainers out on the floor helping people, or do members appear to be wandering around clueless? When you called to make your tour appointment, did the receptionist help you or leave you on hold for ten minutes? Remember, you're never going to be treated any better than before you actually fork over your cash for membership.

It's essential to ask about staff credentials. All professional staff should be certified by a major organization. That's a minimum acceptable standard that, unfortunately, many gyms aren't meeting. For more on this topic, see the "How to Choose a Trainer" sidebar on page 201.

- **The other members.** As closed-minded as it may seem, you should pay attention to the type of person who works out at a particular gym. If it's a gym full of serious bodybuilders and you're simply looking to lose weight, will you feel comfortable sharing the arm curl machine with someone whose biceps are bigger than your thighs? If you don't mind stepping into a different world every time you work out, then this isn't too important a consideration, but I find most people want to see at least a few bodies that closely resemble their own.

- **Offerings.** If you have your heart set on taking spin classes and a gym you're scoping doesn't offer them, think twice before joining. How motivated will you be if your club doesn't have the classes, the equipment, or the staff you really want to use? Think about what's important to you before you go club touring, and cross any gym off your list that does not meet your minimum requirements.

- **Cleanliness and state of repair.** Run—do not walk—away from any facility that seems to be held together by duct tape and fungus. An unclean facility translates into all sorts of icky problems such as athlete's foot, mystery rashes, and chronic colds. While it's okay for a small amount of the equipment to be out of service, there is no excuse for a place that's dirty and in a complete state of disrepair.

- **Terms, extras, cost.** Read the membership contract before you sign on the dotted line so you know what you're paying for. Some gyms have clauses that make it nearly impossible to cancel, while others roll over your membership into a second year without notifying you. Make sure the price you've been quoted covers everything you think it does. If you have to start paying extra for things like group classes and towels, it can quickly add up. Lockers, personal laundry, massage, and personal training are typically not included in the membership.

On a recent trip to Hong Kong I toured many of the gyms on the island. Since Western-style gyms are a relatively new concept there, consumers are not that sophisticated about them. Salespeople take advantage of this by locking people into three-to-five-year memberships that steeply escalate in price each year. Some of the membership prices quoted to me were as high as $10,000 a year for facilities I wouldn't consider joining if they were giving away memberships! Don't get caught in a long-term or lifetime membership trap: You should never, ever purchase a membership for any longer than a year.

Getting in Gear

Because most gyms have such a great selection of cardio machines, I encourage you to try a variety of exercises. Even smaller, stand-alone gyms usually have treadmills, upright bikes, recumbent bikes (where you sit in a seat and pedal out in front of you), bikes with arms, climbers, rowers, and elliptical trainers (a relative newcomer that's sort of a cross between a stair climber and a treadmill). Larger gyms often go further with exotic aerobic gadgets such as skating machines, windsurfing simulators, and stationary kayaks.

Which one of these machines will give you the best heart-strengthening, calorie-burning, fat-melting workout? The one you'll actually use. Whatever you enjoy the most, whatever helps you get your butt in gear day after day is the workout you're most likely to stick with and the one that's most likely to give you the results you're after. For some people that means sticking with their favorite aerobic apparatus workout after workout, but I find most people get better results by rotating through a variety of cardio workout choices, probably because it isn't as boring and you're less likely to develop a repetitive-movement injury.

In general, the principles of how you do your cardio work remain the same regardless of which machine you use. The way you use them depends on your goals:

- If your goal is weight loss, you want to do four to six cardio sessions a week; the majority of these sessions should last for forty-five to sixty minutes, but you should also do one or two shorter, higher-intensity workouts as well. There's some evidence to suggest that tossing in a couple of harder workouts each week helps increase your workout "afterburn." This is when you continue to burn calories at a higher rate than normal even after you've stopped working out. While you always have some afterburn effect from working out, it's quite low and short-lived after an easy workout. Though more research is needed, there is some evidence to suggest that the afterburn of high-intensity workouts lasts for several hours or perhaps even days.

- If your goal is to build speed, power, and muscle, you should do two to five shorter, high-intensity workouts a week with the majority of your time spent doing intervals, sprints, and tempo training (alternating five to fifteen minutes at about 80 percent maximum effort with recovery periods of the same length at about 60 percent effort). You may want to consider "periodizing" your workouts into eight-week cycles: four weeks where you hit your workouts hard followed by four weeks of less strenuous training. This helps cut down on injuries and workout burnout. You'll probably also see faster results because the weeks you rest allow you to build up your reserves for the higher-intensity training weeks. Many top athletes use this type of periodization training.

- If your goal is simply to improve your health, bolster your immunity to disease, and increase stamina, three to six moderately intense workouts a week will do. They can last for as little as twenty minutes and as much as sixty minutes.

- The only time I suggest sticking exclusively to the same cardio workout for long periods of time is if you're training for a specific event such as a marathon, bikeathon, or hiking event. Here a theory called "specificity of training" becomes important. This simply means that if you want to excel at a sport, activity, or event, you train the same way that you compete. For example, if you're a runner, you get better by running. Even then I would still cross-train during your off-season or immediately following your big event.

As for the weight-training equipment you find in the gym, there's plenty of variety there too. The strength-building/body-sculpting workout in this chapter uses weight equipment that's commonly found in the average gym. The primary exercises I've given you utilize weight machines; I've also given you a free-weight alternative for each exercise in case you decide to venture into the free-weight area.

You might be interested to know the difference between machines and free weights. Traditional weight-training machines have fixed-path movements, meaning that when you push or pull on them they can only move in one direction, so you almost can't screw up the movement. This is ideal for novice weight lifters. Weight-training machines have begun to morph in recent years. Some now have paths that are multidirectional or intentionally include a little play in the mechanism so you're forced to use your deep, internal muscles to keep the movement steady.

Free weights consist of metal bars and plates. Barbells are long bars where you usually add and subtract weight plates to get the amount of weight you want to lift for a particular exercise. Dumbbells are shorter and typically come in sets of fixed weights. You pick up the set that corresponds to the weight you want to lift for an exercise. Barbells are ideal for exercises that work both sides of your body in unison, like a Bench Press or Bench Row, whereas dumbbells work each side of your body independently, as with a Fly, an incline Fly, and a One-Arm Row.

Personally, I think both weight machines and free weights have a place in your training. Machines are easier to use, but free weights are more versatile. I think they both do a good job of getting your muscles in shape. The primary workout I've given you in this chapter features machines because they make for a quick, efficient workout, but there is no reason you shouldn't take a mix and match approach.

The Perfect Gym Exercises

As with any type of strength training, it's important to warm up before doing the Perfect Gym Exercises. The Active-Isolated stretches in chapter 10 can serve as a suitable warm-up, as can five to ten minutes of easy-paced activity on any of the cardio machines described in this chapter.

If your priority is losing weight and building stamina, then do your main cardio workout before you do your weights. If strength and sculpting are your main focus, hit the weights first—but again, only after you've properly warmed up. You never want to lift with tight, cold muscles that aren't adequately prepared for the work at hand.

You can do all of the exercises on one day, but alternating a day of upper-body exercises with a day of lower-body and abdominal exercises is also a good way to manage your workouts. Just make sure each muscle group gets worked out at least twice and no more than four times a week and gets at least one day of rest in between workouts. You can also alternate weight lifting and cardio days, at least when you first begin going to the gym, if you find you don't have the energy to do everything on the same day.

Beginners, and anyone whose main goal is to build some strength and tone, should do one set of each exercise, twelve to fifteen repetitions per set, using a weight that's challenging but not the maximum you can lift. Rest thirty to ninety seconds between sets. If you're aiming for serious body sculpting or trying to build size and maximum strength, move on to the intermediate routine once you're ready for more.

Intermediate exercisers should do two or three sets of each exercise, eight to fifteen reps per set. Rest thirty to ninety seconds between sets. This is also the routine you should stick with if your goal is body sculpting and developing moderate amounts of strength. If your goal is building size and serious strength, move on to the advanced routine once you can breeze through the intermediate routine.

Advanced exercisers who are looking to max out size and strength should do three to five sets per exercise, six to eight repetitions per set, using the heaviest weight they can manage while still maintaining good form. Rest for up to three minutes between sets to give your muscles a chance to fully recover so they can give it their best effort in each and every set.

Whichever routine you perform, do the exercises in the order in which they're listed. I've set up the routine to work from the largest upper-body muscles to the smallest. This way, the smaller muscles aren't tired out in the earlier stages and your larger muscles will get a better workout.

You should begin to see noticeable changes in your body after about three to six weeks of consistent workouts. You'll notice that your muscles look firmer, tighter, and shapelier. If you don't have too much body fat, you'll begin to see "cuts," or muscle definition. If you have weight to lose, watch what you eat and keep up regular cardio workouts to drop body fat. You might consider alternating this workout with the Perfect Weight Loss Workout as well.

Real strength gains typically come within six weeks of regular training, although you may find yourself able to lift heavier weights after just a couple of workouts.

■ LEG PRESSES

Muscles Worked: This exercise zeroes in on the muscles of your buttocks and thighs.

Joint Cautions: Mild caution for the knees and lower back.

Starting Position: Before you lie down on the machine, change the settings so that when you lie on your back and your feet rest flat on the footplate, your knees are bent to slightly below a right angle to the footplate. Lie

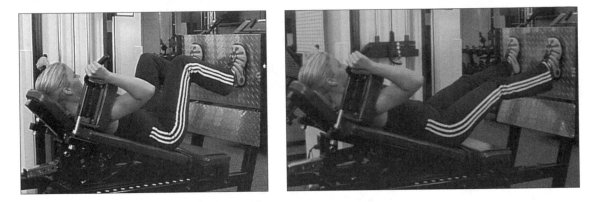

down on the machine with your feet placed hip width apart and your toes pointing forward, heels directly behind your toes. Hold on to the machine's handles and pull your abdominals in.

Exercise: Initiating the movement by pressing through your heels, push upward to straighten your legs. Once your knees are almost but not completely straight, bend your knees to lower toward the starting position. Stop just before the weight stack completely touches down, and move into the next repetition.

Things to Think About:

- At the start of the movement, your body should be positioned as if you're sitting in a chair just slightly too short for you. You'll feel a strong contraction through the front of your thighs as you press upward; some people also feel this exercise in their buttocks.
- Keep your head and shoulders down against the seat pad so that you don't strain your neck.
- It's important not to lock your knees fully at the top of the movement.

Variations:

- **EASIER:** Place your legs a few inches wider than hip width apart and angle your toes slightly outward.
- **HARDER:** To get better isolation of your thighs, place your feet just a few inches apart and don't lower as far.
- **FREE-WEIGHT ALTERNATIVE:** Squats (see description on page 254).

■ LEG CURLS

Muscles Worked: A focused move that isolates the hamstrings.

Joint Cautions: Mild knee caution.

Starting Position: Before you lie down on the machine, place the ankle pads of the machine so that when you lie on your stomach, they line up approximately one inch above your heels. Lie down on the machine with your face turned to the side so you don't strain your neck. Hold on to the handles and flex your feet. Pull your abdominals in and gently press your hip bones downward.

Exercise: Bend your knees until your lower legs are perpendicular to the floor. Hold a moment before lowering to the start.

Things to Think About:
- You'll feel a strong contraction in the center of the back of your thighs, especially when your knees are fully bent at the top of the movement.
- Focus on keeping your hips pressed downward so you get better isolation of the hamstrings.
- Kicking your heels all the way into your buttocks isn't necessary. If you can do it, that probably means the weight is too light or you're moving too quickly.

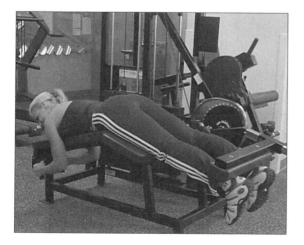
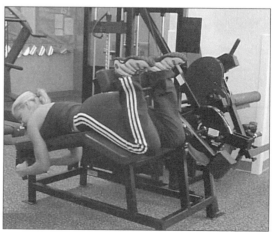

Variations:

- **EASIER:** Many leg curl machines have range-limiting devices that you can set to shorten the arc of the movement. This is a good option if you have very weak hamstrings or if you feel knee pain at any point during the exercise.
- **HARDER:** Lift the weight using both legs but lower with only one.
- **FREE-WEIGHT ALTERNATIVE:** Kneeling Leg Press (see page 49 for details).

■ INNER THIGH MACHINE

Muscles Worked: This machine strengthens and tones the adductor muscles. Many inner thigh machines can also be set to work the outer thighs; if your gym's does, this exercise is a great complement to the inner thigh exercise.

Joint Cautions: None.

Starting Position: Before sitting down on the machine, position the leg and ankle pads so that they are together and rotated to the inside. Sit in the seat so that your knees are bent, your ankles are flush against the ankle pads, and your inner thighs are flush against the thigh pads. Pull your abdominals in and sit up tall.

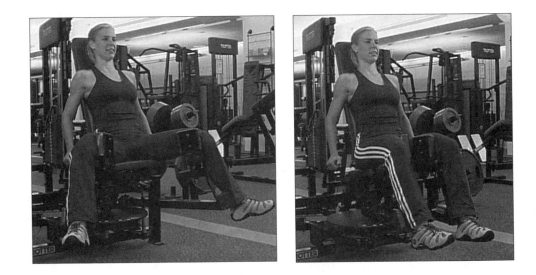

Exercise: Slowly press your legs inward until you feel a strong pull through your inner thighs. Hold a moment and slowly bring your legs outward as far as you comfortably can. Move immediately into the next repetition.

Things to Think About:

- Imagine you are squeezing a heavy object between your legs. You'll feel the strongest pull through the top and inside of your thighs as you hold a moment before returning to the start.

Variations:

- **EASIER:** Many machines enable you to limit the extent of the movement in case you find the full movement too challenging.
- **HARDER:** Hold the innermost part of the movement and do ten small "pulses" before moving inward and beginning the next rep.
- **FREE-WEIGHT ALTERNATIVE:** Inner Thigh Taps (see page 261 for details).

■ MACHINE CALF RAISES

Muscles Worked: This exercise is one of the best calf shapers there is.

Joint Cautions: Slight caution for the knees; neck.

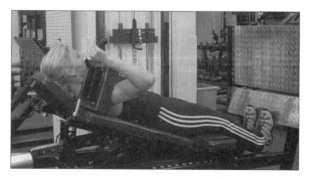

Starting Position: Lie down on the leg press machine with your legs fully straightened and your feet hip width apart, toes pointing forward. Hold on to the machine's handles and pull your abdominals in.

Exercise: Rise onto your tiptoes and lift your heels as high as you can. Hold a moment and then lower your heels past the start, stretching your calves as much as you can before moving into the next rep.

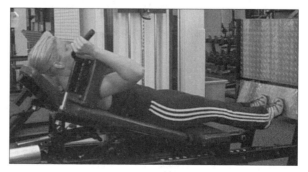

Things to Think About:

- Imagine you are trying to place something on a very high shelf and you need to stand on your tiptoes to reach it. You'll feel a strong pull as you rise upward and a great stretch as you lower.
- To ensure maximum isolation for your calves, keep your knees locked and straight as you do the exercise.
- Avoid arching your back or straining your neck.

Variations:

- **EASIER:** Do not lower your heels below the starting position between reps.
- **HARDER:** Work one leg at a time. Hold the foot of your nonworking leg up off the platform.
- **FREE-WEIGHT ALTERNATIVE:** Toe Raises (see description on page 55).

■ LAT PULL-DOWNS

Muscles Worked: Your upper and middle back are the prime muscles worked with this exercise, but your shoulders and arms get a workout as well.

Joint Cautions: Shoulders, rotator cuff.

Starting Position: Adjust the machine's thigh pads so that when you sit down with your knees bent and your feet flat on the floor, your thighs just above your knees are securely situated underneath the pads. While still standing, grasp the bar with your hands a few inches wider than shoulder width, palms facing forward. Sit down and stretch your arms straight up. Stay tall, keeping your chest lifted. Lean back slightly from your hips.

Exercise: In a smooth, fluid movement, pull the bar down and toward the top of your chest, hold a moment, and then slowly straighten your arms to raise the bar back to the starting position. When you've completed the set, don't let go of the bar until you stand up.

Things to Think About:

- Pulling the bar down toward your chest should resemble a rowing

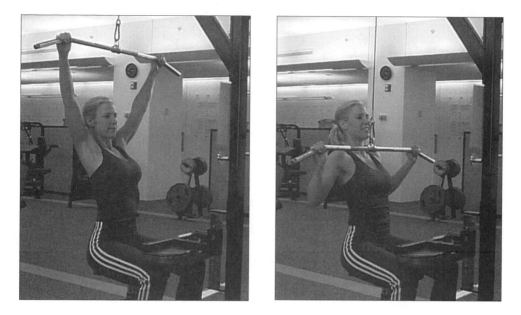

motion. You'll feel this exercise in the outer edges of your upper back as you lower the bar, and you'll feel a great stretch through your arms, shoulders, and the outside of your back as you raise the bar.

- Do control the upward movement of the bar; most injuries from this exercise occur when the bar is raised too quickly.
- Keep your wrists straight or turned slightly forward to ensure that your back muscles are doing the bulk of the work.

Variations:

- **EASIER:** Hold the bar a few inches away from the center with your palms facing in toward you.
- **HARDER:** There are various attachments you can use in place of the long straight bar. A short bar, V-bar, or triangle bar can add a little oomph to this move.
- **FREE-WEIGHT ALTERNATIVE:** Dumbbell Row (see description on page 141).

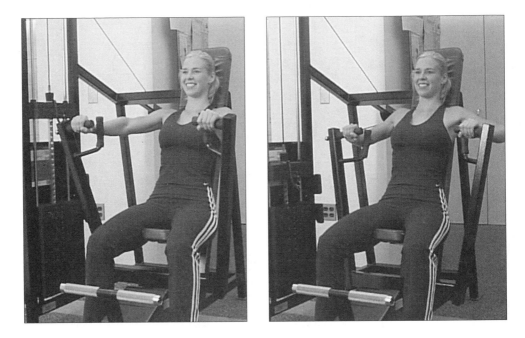

■ CHEST PRESSES

Muscles Worked: This exercise strengthens and tones your chest, shoulders, and triceps.

Joint Cautions: Shoulders, rotator cuff.

Starting Position: Position the seat so that the center of your chest lines up with the center of the horizontal set of handles. (You can usually do this with your butt lifted slightly off the seat; the seat settings are located directly underneath the seat.) Once positioned correctly, sit down in the seat, facing forward, and press down on the foot bar so that the handles move forward. With nearly straightened arms, grip the horizontal handles. Keep your abdominals tight so that your upper back remains on the pad and remove your foot from the foot bar so that all of the weight you are lifting is now transferred to your arms.

Exercise: Bend your arms until your elbows are a few inches behind your shoulders and then press back up to the starting position. Once you've completed the set, place your foot back on the foot bar to transfer the weight back to your foot. Get your arms out of the way as you carefully lower the machine handles.

Things to Think About:

- This is a classic pushing movement; it mimics pushing a heavy object out of your way. You'll feel the back of your arms, center of your shoulders, and middle of your chest working as you straighten your arms; some people also feel muscles contracting as they bend their arms.
- Placing your foot on the foot bar to end the set is very important; if you don't get your arms out of the way, you risk straining your rotator cuff muscles.
- Also important is not bending your arms too far back. This can overstrain your rotator cuff as well.

Variations:

- **EASIER:** Many machines have a range-limiting device to narrow the distance you can move the bar. It's a good idea to use this device if you experience pain at any point during the exercise or if you have a difficult time with this exercise.
- **HARDER:** Use the vertical handles; this isolates your chest muscles more and restricts the involvement of your other muscles.
- **FREE-WEIGHT ALTERNATIVE:** Incline Dumbbell Presses (see page 140 for details).

■ SHOULDER PRESS MACHINE

Muscles Worked: This machine works your shoulders with some help from your arm muscles.

Joint Cautions: Shoulders, elbows.

Starting Position: Set your seat height so that the machine's pulley is even with the middle of your shoulder. (You can usually do this with your butt lifted slightly off the seat; the seat settings are located directly

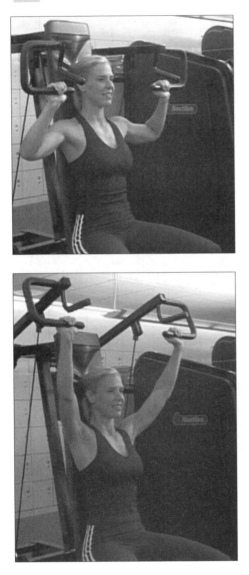

underneath the seat.) Hold on to the front handles with your palms facing each other. Sit up tall, maintaining a slight natural gap between the small of your back and the seat pad.

Exercise: Lift the handles straight up over your head. Straighten your arms until your elbows are slightly bent. Bend your arms to lower the weight until your elbows are just slightly below shoulder height and then move into the next rep.

Things to Think About:

- You'll feel a contraction through the top and center of your shoulders as you press upward. Some people also feel the muscles in the back of their arms working as well.
- Avoid bending your elbows too much between reps; they should move slightly below your shoulder height and no lower.
- Keep your shoulders relaxed and don't over-arch your back to press the weight upward.

Variations:

- **EASIER:** Many machines have a range-limiting device to narrow the distance you can move the bar. It's a good idea to use this device if you experience pain at any point during the exercise or if you have a difficult time with this exercise.
- **HARDER:** Use the vertical handles; this isolates your shoulder muscles more and restricts the involvement of your arms.
- **FREE-WEIGHT ALTERNATIVE:** Military Presses (see description on page 165).

■ CABLE BICEPS CURLS

Muscles Worked: A total biceps isolator.

Joint Cautions: Mild elbow and lower back caution.

Starting Position: Place the cable position all the way at the bottom of the machine's column and attach a short, straight bar. Face toward the column and bend down and grasp the bar a few inches away from the center in an underhand grip. Stand up tall with your feet hip width apart, your arms out straight, elbows in at your sides, abs pulled inward.

Exercise: Bend your elbows and lift the bar up to chest level. Slowly and carefully restraighten your arms to lower to the start.

Things to Think About:

- The strongest contraction you'll feel will be at the center of your upper arm, midway through bending your elbows and lifting the bar up.
- Although your elbows should remain near your sides, avoid actually pressing them into your waist.
- Do not arch backward to lift the weight. If you need to do this, the weight is probably too heavy.

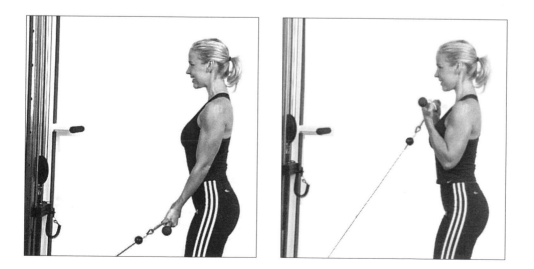

Variations:
- **EASIER:** Place the pulley up one or two notches on the cable frame to limit the amount you can lower the cable.
- **HARDER:** Try this exercise using a V-shaped or W-shaped bar.
- **FREE-WEIGHT ALTERNATIVE:** Basic Biceps Curls (see page 57 for details).

■ CABLE TRICEPS EXTENSIONS

Muscles Worked: A total triceps isolator.

Joint Cautions: Mild elbow, shoulder caution.

Starting Position: Place the cable position all the way to the top of the machine's column and attach a short, straight bar or rope. Grasp the bar a few inches away from the center in a downward-facing grip. Stand up tall about a foot away from the column and facing away from it. Put your feet about a stride's length apart and lean forward from the hips. Raise the bar up and bend your elbows back so that they are on either side of your face, and your hands are level with the top and back of your head.

Exercise: Straighten your arms up over your head to lift the weight.

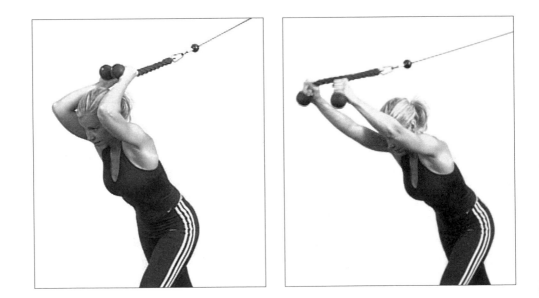

When your arms are nearly but not quite straight, slowly bend your elbows to return to the starting position.

Things to Think About:

- Imagine you're holding an icepick in your hands and trying to hack away at the side of a rock. You'll feel a strong contraction through the entire length of the back of your upper arms as you straighten your arms and press the bar downward.
- Raise the weight up slowly and carefully so you don't snap or strain your elbows.
- Focus on keeping your shoulders relaxed and down and your wrists straight.

Variations:

- **HARDER:** Try this exercise using a V-shaped or W-shaped bar.
- **FREE-WEIGHT ALTERNATIVE:** Basic Triceps Dips (see page 58 for details).

■ HANGING KNEE-UPS

Muscles Worked: A super-focused move for the entire abdominal muscle group.

Joint Cautions: Lower back.

Starting Position: (*Note:* This move can also be done with a captain's chair or high chair if available.) Hang with your upper arms securely placed in two ab straps that are positioned about shoulder width apart. Let your legs hang down and together. Pull your belly button in toward your spine and relax your shoulders.

Exercise: Exhale through your mouth and, keeping your legs together, slowly bend your knees up to your chest. Hold a moment; inhale through your mouth as you slowly lower to the starting position.

Things to Think About:

- When you pull your knees up to your chest, your positioning should resemble a cannonball dive into a pool. You're likely to feel your abdominal muscles working through the entire movement. If you have

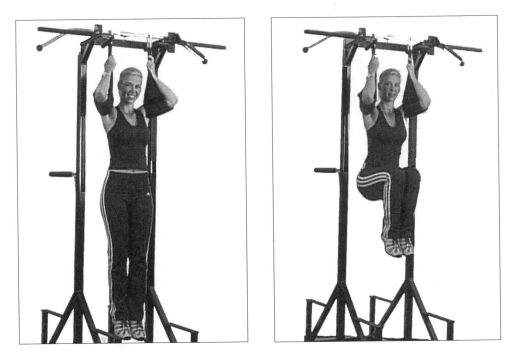

tight hip flexors, you may feel a slight pull at the very top of your thighs as well.

- Focus on keeping your shoulders and neck relaxed so that all of your effort comes from the abdominals.
- Also focus on keeping your abs pulled strongly inward.

Variations:

- **EASIER:** Alternate lifting first the right leg, then the left.
- **HARDER:** You can either hold your knees in the up position for a slow count of five or straighten your legs forward so at the top of the movement, your legs will be closer to an **L** position.
- **FREE-WEIGHT ALTERNATIVE:** Ab Lifts (see description on page 104).

How to Choose a Trainer

Let's say you haven't done anything physical since you climbed the ropes in gym class, or you have a specific goal in mind such as losing weight, or you're curious about what all the little buttons on the treadmill do. These are all good reasons to consider hiring a personal trainer.

A good trainer can help you get in shape quickly and safely. The problem is, there are plenty of bad trainers out there who don't know the difference between a push-up and a push-up bra—and that means a waste of time, energy, and money. Some basic requirements to look for when hiring a personal trainer:

- **A certification from a reputable organization.** There are over 350 fitness-certifying bodies, and unfortunately many of them are questionable. Look for a certification by one of the so-called Big Three: the American College of Sports Medicine, the American Council on Exercise, or the National Strength Conditioning Association. Although I also like to see group fitness instructors certified by ACE, many of the yoga, Pilates, and martial arts teachers have only certifications that apply to their disciplines. These are not standardized, so you'll have to rely on your judgment to evaluate whether an instructor is any good or not.

- **An academic degree in a fitness-related field.** Colleges and universities have bachelor's and master's degree programs that prepare trainers for teaching people how to exercise. Exercise physiology, for example, is the study of the human muscular, skeletal, circulatory, and nervous systems and how they respond to exercise. Exercise physiologists learn how to teach safe exercise to prevent injury and to modify exercise for those who are already injured.

- **Experience.** Has your trainer most recently completed a stint delivering packages for a messenger service? Is she appearing as Rizzo in a regional-theater production of *Grease*? Look for a trainer who has at least two years of steady experience either on her own or in a health club rather than a trainer who is moonlighting as a way to pick up extra cash between gigs.

- **Insurance.** Your trainer must carry liability insurance even if your club also has insurance. There is always a risk you may get injured. A good trainer will be smart enough to have proper insurance coverage for her benefit as well as yours.

- **Personality.** Maybe you prefer the drill sergeant approach, but if you don't and your trainer turns your workout into an episode of *Fear Factor,* it won't inspire you to come back. Decide what training style you prefer and look for a trainer to match it.

Surviving a Group Class

Stepping into a group class for the first time can be pretty intimidating. Pushing your way into prime mirror space is the gym equivalent of fighting over a dress at a bargain-basement sale. And once the music starts, where do your feet go, how are you supposed to swing your arms, and why is everyone else reaching for the toes on their right foot when you're reaching for your left ear? You can survive—even thrive on—the group class experience if you keep these simple guidelines in mind.

- **Choose the right class.** Kickboxing can be one of the greatest workouts going, but wander into a double supersonic, astrophysical martial arts bonanza your first time out and you'll leave feeling confused, sore, and discouraged. If you've never tried a particular type of workout before, peruse the schedule for classes that have the word *beginner* or *basic* in the title.

- **Find your mark.** Choose a place in the classroom where you can easily see the instructor. To avoid the elbowing that occurs as everyone vies for a choice spot, get to the class a few minutes early.

- **Mirror, mirror on the wall.** Does looking in the mirror seem like a reflection of how clumsy you feel as you go through the moves? Readjust your thinking. Use the mirror as a tool to help adjust your body alignment and move correctly.

- **Pass no judgments.** Know this: As a group class neophyte, you *will* make mistakes. It's okay. Allow yourself to be a beginner. And accept that stumbling over your feet a little is just part of the learning process.

- **Don't give up.** Ask the instructor for feedback during and after the class to help speed up your improvement. Even if you're no physical genius starting out, you'll get better. I promise.

Leg Exemption

Sharp readers and seasoned gym goers will notice that there is one piece of equipment commonly found in most gyms that I haven't included in the Perfect Gym Exercises—the leg extension. This is the piece of equipment designed to isolate your quadriceps muscles, the large muscles located in the front of your thighs. The leg extension machine looks like a leather chair with a weight stack welded to it. You sit in it with a pad propped on your ankles and extend your legs straight out to lift the weight stack. So why do I, as well as a growing number of other fitness, medical, and physical rehabilitation experts, recommend avoiding the use of the leg extension?

"When quads contract in isolation under high loads, you expose the knee joint to high levels of sheer stress," warns Cedric Bryant, Ph.D., chief physiologist for the American Council on Exercise in San Diego. "This is a sliding type of stress that causes the bones that reside beneath your kneecap to shift forward, resulting in a lot of wear and tear to the knee joint."

The result is often chronic knee injury and pain. Bryant claims most exercisers are better off skipping leg extensions and sticking to so-called functional exercises such as the squat, leg press, or lunge to work their quads, because these exercises bring the surrounding hamstring and buttocks muscles into the act in much the way your lower-body muscles operate in everyday life. "This offsets any misalignment of the knee," Bryant adds.

According to Bryant, the leg extension can have a place in your training if you specifically want to develop the innermost part of your quadriceps for aesthetic purposes. "You want to limit the range of motion your leg moves through by setting the ankle pad high up on your shin rather than flush with your ankle. This helps reduce sheer stresses placed on your knee," Bryant says.

THE PERFECT STRETCH WORKOUT

Sandra doesn't have a dance or gymnastics background but realized she had the gift of flexibility when she stood on a balance beam with one leg held up in the air during a high-school phys ed class. She got an A in the class, but as she's gotten older she's had to work to maintain her loose and limber limbs. "I find that consistency is the key," she says. "I try to do a little stretching here and there throughout the day." For instance, when she's talking on the phone, she'll stand and do a couple of arm or leg stretches. She also does a more formal flexibility routine at the end of her workouts. Sandra thinks a little bit of stretching offers vast rewards. "You feel more energized and less cranky, plus you look and move better too."

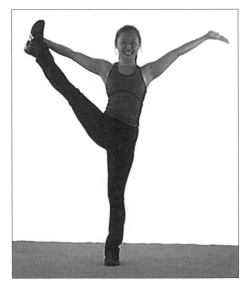

EXERCISES IN THIS CHAPTER

- Shoulder Pendulums
- Backward Reaches
- Alternate Arm Reaches
- Side Neck Stretches

- Single-Arm Side Stretches
- Palm Presses
- Standing Ab/Lower Back Stretches
- Outer Hip Stretches
- Rope Calf Stretches
- Rope Hamstring Stretches

EQUIPMENT NEEDED

- Stretching mat or thick towel
- Stretch rope, belt, or long towel
- A light weight

ESTIMATED WORKOUT TIME

- All levels: 10–15 minutes

My good friend Norman always precedes his daily run by throwing his leg up on the hood of a parked car (not his own, but please don't tell anyone) and grabbing his toes. I've always wondered: Is he stretching his hamstrings properly, or is he simply leaving nasty scuff marks on someone else's paint job?

It's an interesting question, mainly because the answer isn't necessarily what you'd expect. Presumably we reach for our toes or reach for the sky in an effort to prevent injuries, ease muscle soreness, and improve athletic performance. But the truth is, even experts aren't really sure that stretching does any of these things.

For instance, a recent study done at the Physiotherapy Department of the Kapooka Health Centre in New South Wales, Australia, found that stretching did nothing to lower the injury rate of fifteen hundred people who regularly stretched before their workouts. Dozens of other studies have come up with similar findings, and several even found that pre-exercise stretching may actually *cause* injuries.

What about the long-held belief that stretching eases soreness, specifically delayed-onset muscle soreness, the kind of muscle achiness and stiffness that appears twenty-four to forty-eight hours after a workout if you haven't exercised in a while or you've hit the weights harder than usual?

Again, the research says it's not true. And again, some studies found that stretching can often increase soreness, probably because it further traumatizes out-of-shape and overworked muscles.

At least all that preworkout bending and twisting everyone from world-class athletes to weekend warriors has been doing for decades helps you run faster and jump higher, right? Wrong. Or at least possibly wrong. The correlation between better flexibility and superior athletic performance is skimpy at best. And you've probably already guessed what I'm going to say next: Several studies, including a large-scale University of Hawaii study that looked at thousands of runners, found that greater flexibility can have an *adverse* effect on performance due to a sharp increase in injuries.

So is stretching a big waste of time, one piece of the workout puzzle that doesn't fit? Well, since I've devoted an entire chapter to the perfect way to stretch, I think you can safely assume that that is not the case.

Rethinking Stretching

I firmly believe that flexibility is one of the most important aspects of a complete fitness program. We've just got to rethink it.

For starters, the majority of the thirty-five million people who stretch on a consistent basis have been doing so for the misguided reasons I've already debunked above. I think the best motives for stretching are to feel better, look better, and move more comfortably. There is mounting evidence to support the notion that flexibility is a fundamental aspect of fluid movement, better balance, improved coordination, better posture, increased comfort, and deeper relaxation. All of these things impact how you can perform mundane, everyday tasks you hardly give a second thought to, such as walking, stepping off curbs, and bending down to tie your shoelaces.

You only have to look at someone with poor flexibility to see that this is true. Many older people, for instance, tend to shuffle their feet and move with stiff, limited strides; their posture is usually less than ideal, and they're far more prone to falls than younger folks. In part this is due to decreased mobility of their joints. Conversely, those with superior flexibility, such as dancers, gymnasts, and skaters, seem to skim across the floor with grace, ease, and enviable posture. (Note, though, that these three groups of athletes have extremely high injury rates, and some experts speculate that too much flexibility may be a contributing factor.)

I also think that we have been stretching incorrectly, and here's where it gets controversial.

Traditional stretching involves moving into a stretched position and holding it for up to a minute. The idea is to elongate the muscle to as much as 1.6 times its original length. For instance, to stretch the front of your thigh, you might lie on your side and bend your top knee until you can grasp your toe or ankle and hold it there for thirty seconds or more; as you hold, you feel an ever-increasing pull spread from the top of your knee to your hip bone. This is the type of stretching we've been doing for decades, the kind that's been featured in aerobics classes and recommended by fitness trainers—and even doctors—before a workout.

This is also the type of stretching sanctioned by most major fitness organizations, notably the American College of Sports Medicine. The official position of the ACSM recommends daily traditional stretching after a warm-up; they suggest holding each stretch for thirty seconds and doing at least one stretch for every large muscle group in the body.

Now, whenever possible I try to base my opinions on straight science and irrefutable facts. But in this case, I don't think stretching and flexibility have been studied well enough yet. Even the ACSM admits that more research is needed. And even they recommend stretching *after* your workout, when your muscles are warmed up—not before, as most people do—because they recognize that traditional stretching is too harsh for tight, cold muscles. This is why I've stepped away from the party line and why I'm recommending you stretch an entirely different way.

A Different Way to Stretch

Let me tell you about my friend Jane Scott. Jane is a personal trainer who has always been in amazing shape. For the past several years she's been competing in the aerobic champion competitions you seen on ESPN. These competitions favor those with a gymnastic or dance background because you need an exceptional amount of flexibility to be able to do things like jump into the air and land in a full split or kick your leg straight over your head. While Jane has always been stronger than most men I know, she was so inflexible she could barely touch her toes.

With characteristic determination, Jane set out to improve her flexibility by stretching daily for more than an hour a day. I was surprised when I first saw her go through her routine: I expected her to do a lot of conventional stuff, such as hurdler stretches, toe touches, and sustained splits, but instead she seemed to be a blur of movement, doing quick high kicks, leg swings, and arm circles. Curious, I asked her about it.

"I chose to do a lot of dynamic stretching because it allowed me to mimic the sport-specific movements I wanted to be able to do—seated kicks, standing kicks, hip circles—without the risk of injury. This method worked for me because it was aggressive yet comfortable and safe. I can now perform a split with either leg in front, and I know that doing movement-oriented stretches helped me get to this point," she says.

When I thought about it, it made a lot of sense. For the less bendy among us, traditional stretching can be a painful experience, and our muscles may not respond favorably to a lot of sustained tugging and pulling. One possible reason tight muscles may not respond well to a sustained stretch is that when a muscle is stretched too far or too long, it tightens up and springs back upon itself to prevent ripping and tearing. This automatic defense mechanism is known as the myotatic reflex or, less technically, the stretch reflex.

Some experts feel that it's wise to avoid the stretch reflex by keeping the duration of a stretch to a minimum. One such method based on this theory is called Active-Isolated or AI stretching.

AI stretching involves choosing a target muscle, tightening the muscle located on the opposite side of the joint, moving into a brief stretch, and then repeating the entire process about ten times. Let's take that quadriceps muscle again. Using the AI stretch method, you straighten your leg to contract the hamstring (since it's located on the opposite the quadriceps) then immediately bend your knee and hold your ankle for about two seconds to stretch the quad.

Jim and Phil Wharton, a father-and-son exercise science team who own the Wharton Performance Muscular Therapy Clinic in Manhattan, have championed the AI technique for more than a decade. Jim explains why it may work: "Muscles have equal and opposite reactions. When you contract, or shorten, one, the opposite one has no recourse but to relax and lengthen," he says. In other words, when you tighten a muscle located on one side of the joint, the muscle on the other side of the joint must respond by loosening up.

Jim also says that, because the stretches are quick, you sidestep the stretch reflex and, in many cases, the pain and discomfort associated with stretching. I have found this to be true.

The Whartons claim that another advantage of AI is that you're able to isolate one muscle group at a time so you can zero in and stretch it deeply and thoroughly. What's more, you can do AI before your workout as a warm-up because it increases blood flow and body temperature.

My trusted colleague Neal Pire, M.S., agrees. "I think it makes sense. AI is a more comprehensive approach to stretching. While I might argue that static [traditional] stretching will be most adept at addressing postural issues or muscle balance, AI addresses flexibility during movement—when, in my opinion, flexibility is most important. Thus, you can argue that AI is a more functional approach to flexibility," he says. As director of training for Plus One Fitness in New York, Pire has worked with thousands of athletes ranging in ability from world-class to novice. He's had plenty of experience with all different types of stretching, and I value his opinion immensely.

Unfortunately, there isn't much hard-core, scientific confirmation yet to support the Active-Isolated theories, although there are several large, long-term studies in the works. All I can tell you right now is that many of my clients and readers plus an increasing number of experts seem to feel that stretching the active isolated way feels better and gets better results.

Perfect Stretching Tips

The routine in this chapter primarily includes Active-Isolated stretching moves. If you've never done any AI before, this will be a totally different stretching experience. If you avoided stretching—as I have—because you've found it painful and ineffective, keep an open mind and give AI a chance to do its thing. You'll be pleasantly surprised by how painless and easy this routine is to do.

Before you get started, read through the following list of suggestions on how to get the most from stretching. It may take a session or two to understand what you're doing and to get the moves to flow, but be patient. You'll soon be rewarded with improved flexibility and all the advantages that come with it.

- Before you begin this routine, take note of which muscles are tight. Jot down some benchmark information, such as "When I lie on my back and straighten my left leg, I'm about a foot short of being able to completely straighten it to a 90-degree angle." After about three weeks of regular stretching, refer to these notes and make some comparisons. They'll help you gauge any improvements.

- When a stretch calls for you to work each side separately, do all ten stretches with your right side and then ten with your left side. This will give you a deeper, more complete stretch than alternating.

- Do the stretches in the order listed.

- Do one or two sets of each stretch. If one muscle is particularly tight, you can add an extra set.

- You can stretch before your workout as part of a warm-up or after your workout as a cool-down.

- Begin each stretch by moving and contracting the muscle on the opposite side of the joint from the muscle to be stretched; hold the contraction (or tightening) for two seconds and then move into the stretch, holding that position for two seconds as well. This contract-relax sequence helps the targeted muscle prepare and "accept" the stretch. The specific form and technique for each stretch is described in detail within the routine.

- Move from one stretch to another with little or no rest in between. Expect to get a little warm and flushed.

- Never force a stretch or attempt to push a muscle past its natural limit. The maximum stretch should feel somewhere between acute awareness of the muscle and mild discomfort—never outright pain.

- Do this routine nearly every day—twice a day if you feel you want to jump-start your flexibility improvements. You should see and feel real improvements in your flexibility after three weeks of regular stretching. Remember, your flexibility is partially defined by your age, activity level, muscle length, and bone configuration, so don't compare your success to anyone else's. Compare your improvements to where you started.

- Some of the stretches call for the use of a stretching rope. The rope provides leverage, which helps you stretch further. These can be ordered by calling (800) 240–9805. You can substitute a long belt or towel.

- You can learn more about the Whartons' Active-Isolated stretching ideas and routines by visiting their Web site, aistretch.com.

SHOULDER PENDULUMS

Muscles Stretched: A gentle warm-up for your shoulders, back, and arms. This is the only non-Active-Isolated stretch I've included in this chapter. I've included it because it helps alleviate some of the shoulder and rotator cuff pain so many people experience. Notice that even though it isn't an AI stretch, it's still not a passively held movement and therefore is an ideal shoulder-area warm-up.

Joint Cautions: None. In fact, this is a good exercise for those who have chronic shoulder and rotator cuff issues.

Starting Position: Hold a light weight in your left hand and lean forward with your knees slightly bent. Allow your left arm to hang down in front of you, as relaxed as possible. Place your right hand on your thigh for support.

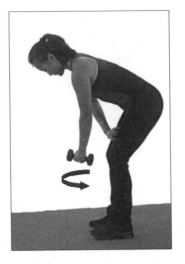

Exercise: Slowly circle your left arm ten times clockwise, then ten times counterclockwise. Don't force the motion; just let it happen. Keep the circles small and well formed. Repeat the movement with your right arm.

Things to Think About:
- Imagine the tight spots in your shoulders as lumps of gravy; the stirring motion of this exercise gently smoothes out those lumps. You'll feel a gentle loosening of your shoulders, upper back, and arms.

Variations:
- **EASIER:** Do one arm at a time. Place your other hand on a table or chair back for support.
- **HARDER:** Increase the weight or increase the number of reps to twenty in each direction.

BACKWARD REACHES

Muscles Stretched: This stretch targets your chest, shoulders, and arms.

Joint Cautions: None.

Starting Position: Stand tall with your feet placed a comfortable distance apart with your arms relaxed down at your sides, palms facing inward.

Exercise: Keeping your elbows straight, reach your arms back behind you as far as you can, hold for one count, and then gently swing your arms to the front of your body at chest level. Reps should be continuous.

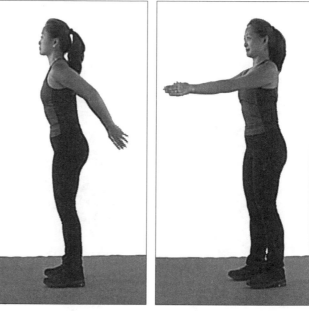

Things to Think About:

• You'll feel a stretch across the top of your chest that should spread through your arms and shoulders with each repetition.

• Resist arching your back each time you reach your arms backward.

• How far you can press your hands back behind you will depend on your flexibility. Your flexibility may not be as great as Sandra's (our model).

Variations:

• **EASIER:** If your flexibility allows, clasp your hands together in back of you and hold each rep for a longer count.

• **HARDER:** Try to raise your arms a little higher in back of you with each successive rep.

◼ ALTERNATE ARM REACHES

Muscles Worked: Shoulders, rotator cuff, chest, upper back.

Joint Cautions: Mild shoulder and rotator cuff caution.

Starting Position: Stand tall with your feet placed a comfortable distance apart. Stretch your right arm up over your head and lengthen your left arm down at your side. Both of your palms should face inward.

Exercise: Keeping your elbows straight and reaching through your

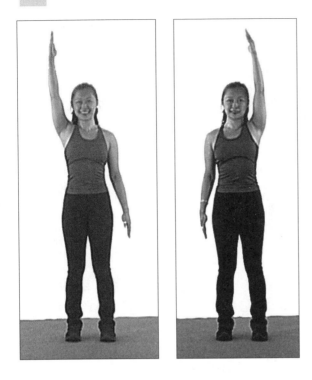

fingertips, extend your right arm up toward the ceiling and your left arm down toward the floor. Hold for one count and then switch arm positions. Keep alternating to complete the set.

Things to Think About:

• Think of your arms as an extension of your back so you feel the stretch not only through your arms and shoulders but also through the entire length of the outer edge of your upper-to-middle back.

Variations:

• **EASIER:** Reach with one arm at a time.
• **HARDER:** Do an additional set with your palms facing forward.

■ SIDE NECK STRETCHES

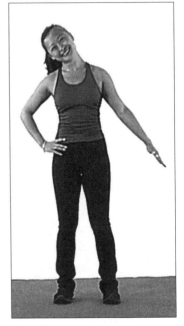

Muscles Stretched: All of the muscles of your neck and tops of your shoulders get a fantastic stretch with this move.

Joint Cautions: Slight neck caution. Use extra care if you're experiencing neck pain.

Starting Position: Stand tall with your feet placed a comfortable distance apart, your left arm down at your side, your right hand on your hip.

Exercise: Cock your head to the side so that your right ear travels toward your right shoulder. At the same time, drop your left shoulder and, stretching through the fingertips, reach your left arm down. Hold for one count and repeat on the other side.

Things to Think About:
- You'll feel a nice elongation of the neck muscles on the opposite side of your neck as you cock your head to the side and hold.

Variations:
- **EASIER:** Do this exercise while sitting.
- **HARDER:** As you cock your head to the right, place your right palm on the top left side of your head and gently assist the stretch.

SINGLE-ARM SIDE STRETCHES

Muscles Stretched: This move stretches the backs of your arms and upper back.

Joint Cautions: None.

Starting Position: Stand tall with your feet placed a comfortable distance apart. Lift your left arm up, bend your elbow, and reach your hand across toward your other shoulder. Place your right hand on the outside of your elbow to gently assist the stretch. Hold a moment.

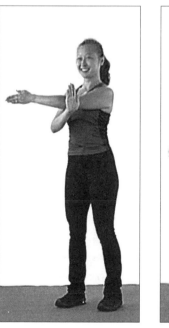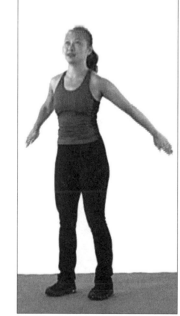

Exercise: Release. Swing your arms back behind you and then repeat to other side. Alternate sides to complete reps.

Things to Think About:
- You'll feel this stretch through the back of your arm and the outer edges of your upper back.

• Try to keep your chin down and avoid jutting your neck forward.

Variations:
• **EASIER:** Don't use your opposite hand to assist the stretch.
• **HARDER:** As you stretch, turn your palm toward your shoulder blade. This will isolate the stretch to the triceps.

■ PALM PRESSES

Muscles Stretched: This wrist stretch is excellent for those who do a lot of typing or repetitive work with their hands.

Joint Cautions: None.

Starting Position: Stand or sit with your left arm extended, palm facing upward.

Exercise: Bend your wrist down and press your right palm against the backs of your fingers to gently assist the stretch. Hold a moment and release. Complete all reps and then repeat to the other side.

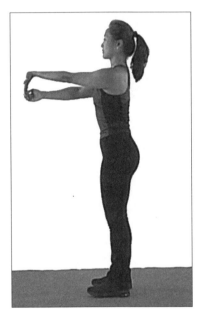

Things to Think About:
• You'll feel an elongation of the muscles in the front of your forearm, especially at the base of your wrist as you press down.

Variations:
• **EASIER:** Do this stretch without pushing on your fingers with the opposite palm.
• **HARDER:** Do another set of stretches where you bend your wrist upward and gently push your hand toward your forearm with your other hand.

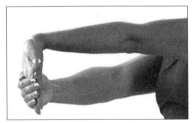

■ STANDING AB/LOWER BACK STRETCHES

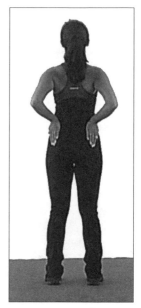

Muscles Stretched: A gentle yet effective stretch for your abs, your lower back, and the tops of your thighs.

Joint Cautions: Mild lower back caution.

Starting Position: Stand with your feet hip width apart. Place your palms on your lower back so that your fingertips extend toward the top of your buttocks.

Exercise: Gently lean back into your palms, pressing your elbows gently behind you. Stretch back far enough to feel a lengthening through your abdominals and a mild tension in the small of your back. Hold a moment. Release and then move into the next stretch.

Things to Think About:
- As I said above, you'll feel a lengthening through your abs and slight tension through your lower back.
- Never force this stretch.

Variations:
- **EASIER:** Lean back a small way without your palms on your back
- **HARDER:** Clasp your hands behind your back and then lean back.

■ OUTER HIP STRETCHES

Muscles Stretched: A deep stretch for the outer hip, top of the thigh, and inner thigh muscles. This is an excellent stretch for those who sit a lot or who experience chronic lower back pain.

Joint Cautions: Mild knee and hip caution.

Starting Position: Sit up tall in a chair with your right foot flat on the floor. Bend your left knee and place the inside ankle on top of your right thigh, just behind your knee. Place your left hand on the side of your knee and your right hand on your hip.

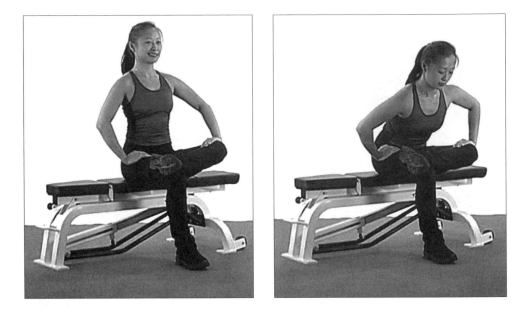

Exercise: Gently press down on your knee with your left hand. Hold a moment and release before moving into the next rep. Do all reps on the right side and repeat with your right leg.

Things to Think About:
- You'll feel a deep stretch through your thighs and hips, especially the inner thigh and outside of the hips, as you press down.
- Try to press your thigh as close to flat as possible, but don't force the stretch.

Variations:
- **EASIER:** Place a rolled-up towel underneath your ankle.
- **HARDER:** Lean a small way forward as you press down on your knee.

■ ROPE CALF STRETCHES

Muscles Stretched: All of the muscles in your calves.

Joint Cautions: None.

Starting Position: Hold a stretching rope or towel as you sit on the floor with both legs stretched out in front of you. Loop the center of the rope around the instep of your right foot and hold an end in each hand.

Exercise: Flex your foot toward you as you gently use the rope to assist the stretch. Hold a moment and then point your toes without resisting with the rope before moving into the next rep. Complete all reps with your right ankle and then repeat with your left.

Things to Think About:
• You'll feel a strong stretch through your calves as you flex your foot.
• Concentrate on keeping your ankle in line with the rest of your calf.

Variations:
• **EASIER:** Do this exercise without the rope.
• **HARDER:** Do this stretch with your leg held a few inches off the floor. This will kick in your hamstring muscles as well, especially if you lean forward slightly.

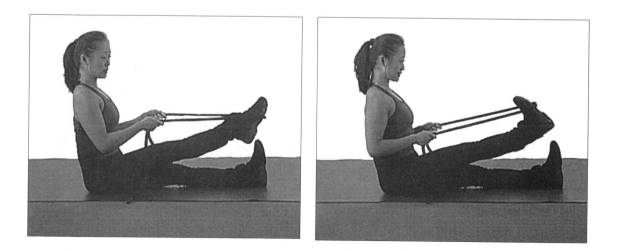

■ ROPE HAMSTRING STRETCHES

Muscles Stretched: This is an excellent isolation stretch for the hamstrings.

Joint Cautions: Mild lower back caution.

Starting Position: While holding a rope or a towel, lie on the floor. Loop the rope around the instep of your right foot and grasp the ends of the rope in your right hand. Bend your left leg and place your foot flat on the floor; lift your right leg off the floor and bend your knee so that your lower leg is parallel to the floor.

Exercise: Straighten your right leg up to the ceiling and, once it is straight, gently pull downward on the rope to increase the stretch. Hold a moment and return to the starting position. Complete all reps with your right leg and then repeat with your left.

Things to Think About:

- You'll feel a gentle yet intense stretch spread through the back of your thigh as you straighten your leg and pull down on the rope.
- To avoid overstretching, don't use the rope to help straighten your leg. Wait until your leg is straight and then use the rope for assistance.
- Keep your lower back and buttocks on the floor.

Variations:

- **EASIER:** Straighten your leg at hip level instead of pointing it to the ceiling.
- **HARDER:** Keep your left leg straight as you stretch the right leg, and vice versa.

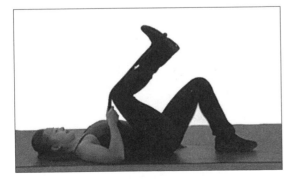 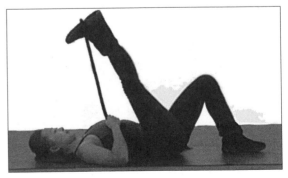

Bending, the Truth

Does stretching really elongate your muscles and make you taller? This is a commonly asked question. The answer is yes and no. "Stretching won't turn you into a giant if you're petite," says Jim Wharton, "but it will allow you to stand up to your full anatomical height." According to Wharton, tight muscles develop adhesions, weblike structures that compress and shorten muscle fibers. (A weight lifter who builds layer upon layer of thick, bunchy muscles is a perfect example of a strong yet tight body.)

"Stretching helps break up those adhesions so muscles can lengthen," he claims. This improves posture, allowing you to stand up straighter so you appear to have gained height.

Wharton says most people will appear to have noticeably longer limbs after a week or so of consistent stretching. "But if you don't continue to work on your flexibility on a regular basis, you lose it," he warns.

Mind-Body Flexibility

Active-Isolated is by no means the only alternative flexibility enhancement technique. Here are some other interesting programs you may want to check into. All four ask your mind to participate in helping put more bend in your body. For more mind-body exercise ideas, flip to chapter 11.

- **Feldenkrais:** Through hundreds of simple exercises that involve visualizing a movement as well as actually doing the movement, Feldenkrais increases awareness of how you use your body so you can progress closer to ideal movement patterns, with improved flexibility and greater strength. Most exercises involve no special equipment. You can do these exercises on your own or with a certified Feldenkrais instructor (www.feldenkrais.com).

- **Alexander Technique:** By making subtle adjustments to everyday movements such as the way you stand or walk, this technique teaches you to let go of unnecessary muscle tension. Easing tension restores natural flexibility and alignment. Look for small group class at the gym or individual instruction. I admit I've tried Alexander and didn't get much out of it, but I know a lot of people who swear by it (www.alexandertechnique.com/at.htm).

- **Hellerwork:** During a private Hellerwork session, a trained therapist combines deep-tissue massage with emotional awareness and movement education. It's aimed at stretching and realigning your fascia, the soft connective tissue that intertwines with the muscles all over your body, so that you can move about more easily (www.hellerwork.com).

- **Trager:** A system of effortless movements to enhance the body's sense of lightness, freedom, and flexibility. Rhythmic massage and stretching encourage the body to let go. Movements involve swinging, stretching, pressing, and rocking the entire torso, as well as meditation and other relaxation strategies (www.trager.com).

THE PERFECT MIND-BODY WORKOUT

Lainey Tant is a rare yoga instructor: besides extensive training in several mind-body disciplines, including yoga, the Alexander Technique, and Polarity, she is also certified through mainstream fitness organizations such as the American Council on Exercise and the American College of Sports Medicine. She's been teaching yoga privately and to groups for more than eight years and helped design the exercises in this chapter. "With mind-body exercises you're able to access a deeper, more integrated aspect of yourself," she says. "You learn to tap into a wellspring of energy and often experience a sense of joy and accomplishment." Lainey believes in the physical benefits of mind-body work as well. She says it's a gentle way to improve strength, flexibility, and posture.

EXERCISES IN THIS CHAPTER

- Chair Pose
- Standing Seat
- Greeting the Sun
- Downward-Facing Dog
- Cat-Cow
- Bird Dog

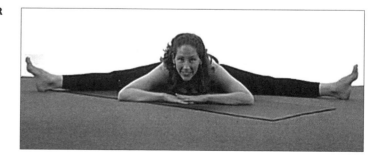

- Mother-Father Earth
- Child's Pose
- Cobra
- Crocodile Pose

EQUIPMENT NEEDED

- Exercise mat or thick towel

ESTIMATED TIME NEEDED

- To start: 15–20 minutes, twice a week
- As you advance: 25–30 minutes, twice a week

Jennifer, a twenty-six-year-old research scientist from Maryland, has been practicing yoga for about two years. She began as a way of escaping the stress of planning her wedding but found that she enjoyed it so much, she's continued with daily yoga sessions ever since.

"One of the major problems I have with some people talking about yoga as their form of exercise is that they only refer to it as a 'workout.' Yoga is much more than an exercise regime; it's more of a lifestyle. Much of my daily life, not just how I exercise, is affected by yoga," Jennifer says.

Jennifer is not alone in this way of thinking. Yoga has its share of dedicated disciples who believe as much in its spiritual benefits as they do in its physical advantages. In other words, they believe that the mind and the body are integrally connected and that each profits from the full participation of the other.

Yoga is one branch of what's come to be known as mind-body exercise. The idea that your mind can make a contribution to exercise has been accepted by a lot of the world, especially in the Eastern cultures, for more than five thousand years but has only recently gained credence in mainstream America. Until about five years ago most exercisers were too busy pumping iron or pounding the pavement to pay much attention to this concept. Oh, sure, you might pass by the occasional yoga class in your gym and make note of the dimmed lights and mysterious chanting. Perhaps you even felt a slight tug of curiosity. But you probably wondered, "Is it exercise? Is it a waste to spend time on something that doesn't seem to cause a calorie to burn or a muscle to firm?"

"What I find great about yoga is that I don't have to jump around like someone with St. Vitius's disease doing aerobics, nor run the risk of tearing and straining something with weight lifting. If I listen to my body, my practice is safe," states aStarseeker, one of the "community leaders" of the yoga board on iVillage.com.

aStarseeker's statement sums up one of the main reasons for the popularity of the mind-body phenomenon: As the population ages and bodies start to deteriorate from decades of joint-crunching activities, more and more people are looking for something "safe" to do. They're looking for exercise that goes beyond heavy sweating and throwing off calories. They're looking for a way to chill out and take a break from the world while getting in better touch with their bodies.

Stress reduction is another fringe benefit of mind-body exercise. "I find myself more centered and relaxed as a result of yoga, not just after I practice, but during the day. When I'm at my day job and I feel overwhelmed," Jennifer says, "I do some breathing exercises and that calms me. It isn't meditation per se, but more of a mechanism to bring me back to myself." Practitioners of Tai Chi, Pilates, and other forms of mind-body exercise often echo the same sentiments.

Personally, I think the mind-body connection is a great development in the fitness evolution. However, I think these mind-body concepts can apply to exercise across the board. I believe that when you bring your brain along with you and fully engage it, aerobics becomes more than simply jumping around, and weight training ceases to put you at high risk for tearing and straining. You add an element of relaxation, learn to clean up sloppy body mechanics, and prevent injuries.

I've attempted to share this belief with you by including hints and suggestions throughout this book on how to make every moment of exercise into a mind-body experience. Notice the "Things to Think About" section I've included within every exercise description in every exercise chapter.

Physical Benefits

Lest I give you the impression that mind-body exercise is only about soul-searching and getting to know your muscles better, let me assure you that it also has many physical benefits as well.

YOGA

Yoga, regardless of which style you practice, does a good job of improving flexibility and building moderate amounts of strength. There is a tremendous focus on proper breathing, posture, and body alignment. Some yoga styles offer more of what I like to call the "golden ball of light factor," so named for the chanting, imagery, and amount of spiritual commitment they require. Studies show that a high "golden ball of light factor" can have positive effects on stress reduction and can lower resting heart rate and blood pressure. (Okay, so scientists don't use this exact phrase, but the ideas they examine are the same.) However, some of the more challenging yoga styles, especially those done in extreme heat, have been shown to increase blood pressure as much as walking on a treadmill at a moderate pace, so if you have high blood pressure, check with your doctor before beginning this type of program.

PILATES

Although it sounds like one of those $8 coffee drinks they sell at Starbucks, Pilates is in fact another highly sophisticated exercise form. It's an exercise technique invented about a century ago by an ex-carpenter and gymnast, Joseph Pilates, to help heal injured war veterans and dancers. There are two ways to practice Pilates (pronounced pih-LAH-tees). You can take a group class on a mat, where you'll do specialized calisthenics exercises, or you can take private lessons on a series of specially designed machines with names like the Cadillac and the Reformer.

Whether you take the mat class or use the machines, all Pilates moves are designed to work your powerhouse muscles—abs, lower back, thighs, and buttocks—and to teach you proper alignment so you move more freely and gracefully. Nothing is forced or repetitive; you emphasize correct form rather than going for the burn. Pilates increases strength, flexibility, and endurance; improves posture, alignment, coordination, and balance; and, on the medical front, has been found to be beneficial in knee and lower back rehabilitation.

TAI CHI

In New York's Chinatown, many older Chinese men and women gather near the waterfront early in the morning to practice tai chi. They move through slow, gentle choreographed movements that resemble swimming underwater. It's beautiful and calming to watch.

While it may not seem like much in the way of exercise, tai chi offers a surprising array of physical payoffs. Numerous studies, including several published in major medical journals such as the *Journal of the American Medical Association* and the *New England Journal of Medicine*, have reported improved flexibility and strength, increased stamina, better posture, reduced hypertension, and more efficient heart function as a result of regular tai chi practice. (It's probably the most completely studied and best-understood of the mind-body techniques.)

OTHER MIND-BODY TECHNIQUES

There are many other less well known disciplines that also have value. NIA, short for the overly technical term Neuromuscular Integration Action, is a series of dance-based movements that increase freedom of movement and reduce pain. The Alexander technique reeducates ingrained body movement patterns through touch and a series of simple exercises. Qi gong (pronounced SHE-gong) uses breath, tai chi–like movements, and meditation to promote relaxation, strength, and flexibility. If you're interested in exploring, there's plenty of information on the Web.

MIND-BODY TECHNIQUES AND WEIGHT LOSS

Before we move on to other topics, I do want to address one last commonly asked question about yoga, Pilates, and other mind-body exercise regimens: Will they help you lose weight?

"Yoga is suddenly being touted as the magic weight loss method. The American media have jumped on this concept and are misrepresenting it badly. Yoga is *not* a weight loss method. Those believing the media will become discouraged and move on before any other yogic benefits are felt," aStarseeker astutely observes.

I agree with aStarseeker. Despite the many wonderful gifts these activities offer, weight loss is probably not one of them. Most forms of mind-body exercise were never intended to be used as a primary calorie-burning, heart-pumping weight loss activity, and there is no scientific evidence that they work this way.

Mind-Body Tips

As you are reading this, is your back hunched over? Are your shoulders tight? Is your head tilted to one side? Stop. Take a deep breath and fix your body. Feel better? Look better? There, you've just made a mind-body connection. You've tuned into how body positioning can make a big difference in how you look and feel.

Making simple adjustments to your body positioning is just one way you can use the idea of the mind-body connection to improve how you sit, stand, and move. Here's a rundown on some others:

- **Meditation, imagery, and visualization.** High-level athletes have been using mindfulness techniques for years. They often visualize themselves winning an event or successfully completing a world-record effort in their mind's eye before the actual event. Though you're probably not attempting world-class physical feats, you can use imagery to help make exercise easier. For instance, as you're walking up a hill, you might imagine a rope. You cast your imaginary rope around an imaginary fence post a few yards ahead of you and use it to help pull you onward and upward.

- **Self-talk.** Whether you know it or not, you've got an internal dialogue going on all of the time, even when you exercise. That voice is often negative. It may tell you that you're not strong enough to lift a weight or that you'll never be able to tone your arms. That voice is also under your control. You can practice a sort of affirmation before your workout and even while you're going through it. The more often you can tell yourself you can achieve your goals, the more likely you are to believe in yourself and achieve them.

- **Body awareness.** Tuning into what your body is experiencing during a workout can be very enlightening. (Want a big word for this? Experts refer to body awareness as proprioception or kinesthetic awareness.) Based on the feedback your body sends to your brain, you can make instantaneous adjustments and take note of how your body responds to specific circumstances for future reference. For example, during a run or walk you can progress through a head-to-toe checklist of your body, taking note of how each part of your body feels and how it is responding. If you have, say, a tendency to shuffle along, you can remind yourself to loosen up your hips, lift your knees, and lengthen your stride. (You can find a sample checklist on page 63.)

- **Breathing.** I could write an entire book on how to breathe and the meditative, relaxing and energizing benefits of proper breathing. Indeed, entire books *have* been written on this topic. Suffice to say that I've given you proper breathing cues through this book. In traditional weight training, you exhale when you're exerting an effort and inhale when you're releasing the effort; in yoga, Pilates, the moves in this chapter, and other types of mind-body exercise, mindful breathing is often the primary reason for doing the move.

- **Posture and alignment.** One of my favorite aspects of taking a mind-body approach to exercise is that you learn to pay attention to how your body looks. This is not narcissistic. When you take note that your head is pressed too far forward or that your shoulders are hunched up toward your ears, you can make corrections that very likely will save you from injury or at least discomfort. So go ahead and look in the mirror while you're lifting weights or practicing yoga. It will give you instant insight into some things you should change.

- **Energy flow.** *Vital life force*, *chi*, and *prana* are just a few terms used to describe the flow of energy you feel when your body is in movement. In some mind-body disciplines, learning how to control your energy is the main event. I believe that the concept of energy control can be applied to virtually any activity you do, whether it's pressing your *chi* into a ball, as you do in tai chi, or knowing when to gather yourself for that extra burst of effort when lifting a weight.

These techniques may have their roots in Eastern philosophy, but there is no reason you can't apply them to everything you do in the name of exercise. They're just as useful to get the most from weight lifting, running, riding your bike, and striding on the elliptical trainer as they are in yoga and Pilates. Use them when you do the exercises in this chapter—and with all of the exercises in this book, for that matter.

The Perfect Mind-Body Exercises

The routine that follows contains moves, or postures, inspired by a variety of mind-body disciplines. It includes many yoga moves, but strictly speaking it isn't a yoga routine, so it probably won't satisfy the yoga purist. I've borrowed moves from yoga, Pilates, and other Eastern-influenced exercise forms to create a routine that I think you will find a good introduction to the mind-body experience.

You can do this routine every day if you want, but for best results I recommend performing it at least twice a week. Do one to three sets of each move, one to four repetitions per move. If a move is bilateral (you work each side of your body separately), do an equal number of repetitions on each side. All of the exercises should be suitable for all level of exercisers; try the suggested variations if you need to adjust the difficulty.

If you don't like the stretch routine in "The Perfect Stretch Workout," chapter 10, this group of postures is a suitable substitute. Because these moves aren't harsh and won't result in a major tug-of-war with your muscles, you can do them as a warm-up before a cardio or weight-training workout. They also make an ideal cool-down or stand-alone workout you can do whenever you want to relax.

You should see results in the form of increased flexibility, moderate strength gains, and taller posture in about a month. You'll feel the calming effects immediately.

■ CHAIR POSE

Benefits: A wonderful way to improve posture, lengthen your spine, and get a head-to-toe stretch, this pose also offers strength benefits for the legs, abs, and pelvic muscles.

Joint Cautions: None.

Starting Posture: With a long spine and with your feet together, lean slightly forward at the hips and raise your arms overhead.

End Posture: Bend your knees a few inches and press your legs together as you press your palms together and lengthen your arms upward as far as you comfortably can. Breathe deeply as you hold for a few minutes.

Things to Think About:

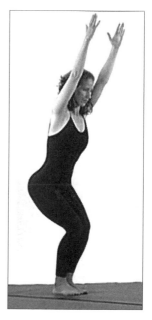

- Think of stretching your fingertips up to the ceiling as you press your feet into the floor. You'll feel a powerful stretch through your entire spine all the way up through your arms. You'll also feel your lower-body muscles working.
- Keep your eyes forward to help align your entire spine, including your neck.
- Keep your spine naturally aligned; don't arch your lower back or tuck your pelvis under.

Variations:
- **EASIER:** Do this move from a kneeling position.
- **HARDER:** Do this move while in a low squat. You may place a rolled-up mat or towel under your heels to aid with flexibility and balance.

■ STANDING SEAT

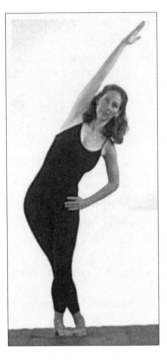

Benefits: This posture provides a deep stretch for your outer hips and buttocks. It offers moderate strength benefits for your lower-body muscles.

Joint Cautions: Mild knee caution.

Starting Posture: Stand tall with your left leg crossed over your right. Press both legs firmly together. Place your left hand on your hip and lift your right arm upward.

End Posture: Bend your knees and "sink into" your hips. Reach your right arm over your head and to the left. Hold a moment and repeat to the other side.

Things to Think About:
- As you sink into your hips you should feel strong and stable. You'll feel a stretch in the outside of your right hip. The longer you hold the posture the more you'll feel a lengthening through your entire right side up into your fingertips.
- Remember to inhale and exhale as you hold the posture.
- Your flexibility may not be as great as Lainey's, our model.

Variations:
- **EASIER:** If you can't find stability in this stance, hold on to a chair for support.
- **HARDER:** Stretch both arms up and out to the side.

■ GREETING THE SUN

Benefits: A pose that helps properly align the pelvis and stretches the tops and fronts of your thighs, your entire torso, and your arms. Calms the mind and promotes a deep sense of relaxation.

Joint Cautions: None.

Starting Posture: Bring your left leg forward so that your knee is bent, your foot is flat on the floor, and your thigh is parallel to the floor. Extend your right leg behind you.

End Posture: Extend your arms straight upward with your palms facing inward. Pull your abdominals gently inward and keep your shoulders down and back. Stretch upward as you shift your weight slightly forward onto your front leg.

Things to Think About:

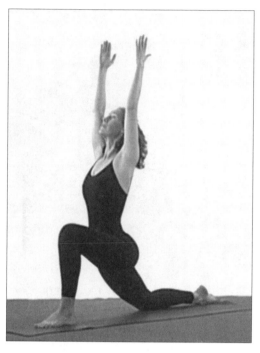

- Think of stretching your fingertips up toward a warm and inviting sun. You'll feel an elongation of your spine and arms as you stretch upward; you'll also feel a gradually increasing stretch through the back of your right thigh as well. Some people feel a tightness in the top of the front part of the thigh.

Variations:

- **EASIER:** Place your hands on the front of your thigh for better balance.

DOWNWARD-FACING DOG

Benefits: This is an intense stretch for your hamstrings, spine, and arms. It releases your body's tension and promotes balance.

Joint Cautions: Lower back, knees.

Starting Posture: Get down on your hands and knees, making sure that your hands are directly under your shoulders and your knees are directly beneath your hips. Pull your belly button in toward your spine and tuck your chin toward your chest.

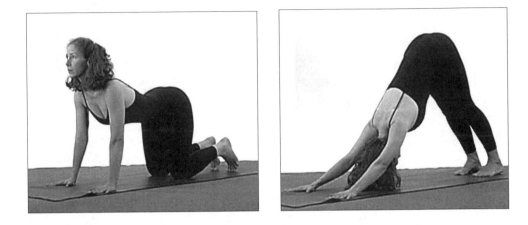

End Posture: Arch your back slightly and then press your body back-ward so that your arms and legs straighten, your tailbone lifts up in the air, and your chest presses toward your thighs. Do your best to press your palms and the soles of your feet into the floor. Hold this position for several moments as you breathe deeply, then move back to the starting position.

Things to Think About:
- In the final position, your body will form an inverted V and your hands will be out in front of your body. You will feel a strong pull through the backs of your thighs. Some people will also feel this deep stretch all the way through the back and into the arms.
- Stretch to your point of comfort. Never force yourself further than you feel comfortable.

Variations:
- **EASIER:** Bend your knees as much as you need to and lift your heels off the floor a small way. If this pose is still too difficult, place your hands on a box or the seat of a chair.
- **HARDER:** Stretch one of your legs up in the air as high as you can.

■ CAT-COW

Benefits: This posture offers a gentle way to stretch the spine and strengthen the abdominals and lower back. It relaxes the mind and eases muscle tension.

Joint Cautions: Mild lower back caution.

Starting Posture: Get down on your hands and knees, making sure that your hands are directly under your shoulders and your knees are directly beneath your hips. Pull your belly button in toward your spine and tuck your chin toward your chest.

End Posture: Exhale, contract your abdominals, and tuck your pelvis under to arch your back upward and drop your head toward the floor. Hold a moment, then inhale, relax your abdominals, and lift your buttocks upward to arch your back downward; lift your head upward. Hold a moment and then continue arching upward and downward without resting between repetitions.

Things to Think About:
• This exercise is so named because as you arch your back up you resemble a Halloween cat and as you arch your back down you resemble the posture of an old cow. You'll feel a general loosening of the spine.

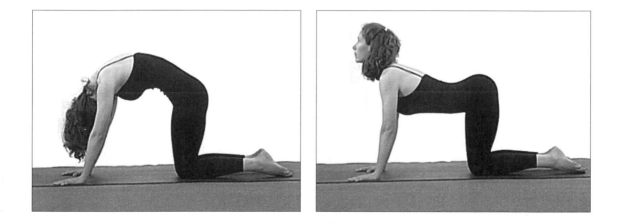

Variations:
- **EASIER:** If either direction of arching bothers you, skip it and just return to the "neutral" position before moving into the next rep.
- **HARDER:** Try the Active Cat exercise described on page 259.

■ BIRD DOG

Benefits: This is the perfect awareness posture to strengthen and stretch your lower back and align your spine. It also helps you master balance and provides moderate strengthening benefits for your arms and legs.

Joint Cautions: None.

Beginning Posture: Get down on your hands and knees, making sure that your hands are directly under your shoulders and your knees are directly beneath your hips. Pull your belly button in toward your spine and tuck your chin toward your chest.

End Posture: Stretch your left arm out at shoulder height, palm facing down, as you extend your right leg out at hip height. Focus on staying as long and relaxed as you possibly can. Hold for a slow count of ten and then repeat with your right arm and left leg.

Things to Think About:
- Stretch through your fingertips and toes, imagining you are trying to

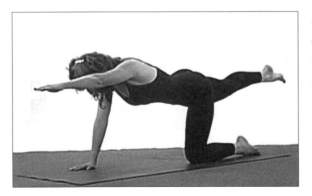

touch the nearest wall. You'll feel a wonderful stretch through the entire length of your spine, arm, and leg. You'll also feel your supporting leg and arm working to keep you in balance.
- Your arms and legs should form a box that resides directly beneath your hips and shoulders.
- Breathe slowly and deeply as you hold the extended position.

Variations:

- **EASIER:** Separate the arm and leg extension into two separate movements.
- **HARDER:** Instead of being on hands and knees, lie on the floor. This will challenge your lower back muscles quite a bit more.

■ MOTHER-FATHER EARTH

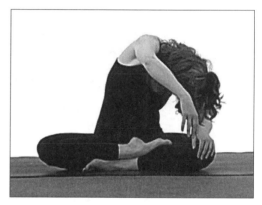

Benefits: Besides having a total calming effect, this pose provides a gentle stretch for the entire spine, shoulders, and arms.

Joint Cautions: Mild lower back caution.

Starting Posture: Sit up tall with one leg crossed over the other. Relax your arms and rest them on top of your legs.

End Posture: Take a deep breath, round forward, and reach your right arm up and over, slightly to the left. Exhale and hold a moment. Return to the start and repeat to the other side.

Things to Think About:

- Imagine that you are reaching up and over a large, soft ball. You'll feel a gentle elongation travel up your spine, through your uplifted arm, and into your fingertips.
- Pull your abs gently into your spine to protect your lower back.

Variations:

- **EASIER:** Round forward without lifting your arm.
- **HARDER:** As you round, reach both arms up and to the side.

■ CHILD'S POSE

Benefits: Eases lower back tension, stretches the spine, quiets the mind.

Joint Cautions: None.

Starting Posture: Kneel on the floor and then sit back so that your buttocks are resting on your heels.

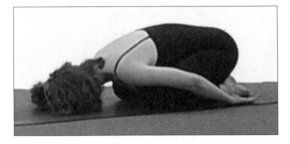

End Posture: Keeping your spine long yet relaxed, bend forward from the hips until your forehead touches the floor and your chest rests on top of your thighs. Relax your arms along your sides. Inhale and exhale deeply and slowly, feeling the motion of your rib cage rise and fall.

Things to Think About:
- You'll feel a deep sense of relaxation gradually come upon you as you hold this posture. Any tension in your spine should ease.
- If you lack flexibility, you may not be able to keep your buttocks on your heels as you stretch forward.

Variations:
- EASIER: Spread your knees apart slightly and place a small cushion under your ankles.
- HARDER: Stretch your arms out in front of you, palms facing upward.

■ COBRA

Benefits: This posture refreshes your body as it relaxes your mind. It opens the chest, stretches the abdominals, and strengthens the upper back, lower back, buttocks, and thighs.

Joint Cautions: Lower back.

Starting Posture: Lie on your stomach with your legs out straight and together and your forehead on the floor. With your elbows bent several inches, place your hands on the floor a little in front and to the sides of your shoulders. Press your palms into the floor and lift your chest a small way off the floor.

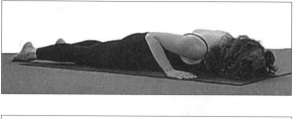

End Posture: Engaging your back muscles, press your palms even more firmly into the floor to straighten your arms and raise your upper body off the floor. Press upward only as much as you feel comfortable. Hold a moment and then slowly lower to the starting position.

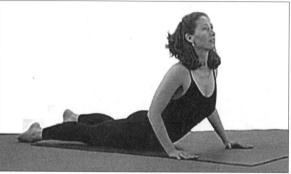

Things to Think About:

- You'll feel a tightening in your lower back and buttocks and a stretch in your abdominals. You'll also feel your arms working to hold your body off the floor.
- How far upward you can press depends on your flexibility and lower back strength. Never force this posture to the point of pain.
- Make sure your hip bones remain on the floor throughout.

Variations:

- **EASIER:** Place your forearms on the floor and press up off them rather than your palms.
- **HARDER:** Stretch your arms out in front of you and lift your upper body, including your arms, up off the floor. Keep your legs down and pressed together with your buttocks muscles engaged to protect your lower back.

■ CROCODILE POSE

Benefits: A wonderful position to help you relax and breathe deeply.

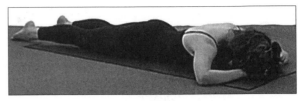

Joint Cautions: None.

Starting Posture: Lie on the floor with your forehead resting on your folded arms so that your chest is elevated slightly off the floor. Stretch your legs out behind you and separate them a comfortable distance with your toes turned outward.

End Posture: Close your eyes and focus on relaxing every part of your body. Breathe deeply and regularly, in and out, for fifteen slow breaths.

Things to Think About:
- Imagine that each breath cleanses your body. The longer you hold this pose, the more relaxed and aware of your body you'll feel.

Variations:
- **EASIER:** Place pillows underneath your hips or any other area of your body you have trouble relaxing or making comfortable.

Lotus Notes

My hard-core yoga friends, readers, and clients tell me that the best way to get into yoga is to find a studio that specializes in yoga. If the yoga classes at your gym are the only option, make sure you choose a teacher who is dedicated to the "yoga lifestyle" as opposed to someone who has acquired a certification over the weekend.

There are as many different types of yoga as there are flavors of yogurt. Which one is right for you? This primer provides a thumbnail sketch of the most popular yoga styles.

- **Hatha:** Because it is the most basic and straightforward of all the styles, most beginning yoga classes are Hatha. The moves flow from standing to seated, with an emphasis on breathing and relaxation. Hatha is the most accessible, least meditative style of yoga.

- **Kundalini:** Consists mainly of seated breathing exercises and chanting "*sat nam,*" a mantra that translates to "truth is my identity." The purpose of this is to relieve stress and calm the mind. The word *kundalini,* by the way, means "energy."

- **Bikram:** This is a hard-core yoga approach: It's done in a room heated to 100 degrees based on the theory that high temperatures make muscles warmer and more pliable. The poses, held for up to one minute, require a combination of flexibility and strength. Needless to say, Bikram is not a good choice for beginners or those who just want to dabble.

- **Iyengar:** Emphasis is on flexibility and alignment. Props such as belts, blocks, and blankets help you push the postures further and increase precision. Good for the athletically minded who don't like to stretch on their own.

- **Ashtanga:** This is another yoga style that works well for athletes and conventional exercisers because it promotes flexibility, stamina, and strength. Many so-called power yoga classes are Ashtanga-based.

Thinking Thin Thoughts

Is it possible that losing weight is all in your head? Absolutely, according to sports psychologist Shane Murphy, Ph.D., assistant professor of psychology at Western Connecticut University. "If you're trying to get motivated to lose weight, you need to have a long-term goal. To the extent you can picture that, make it real, believe that it's really going to happen—it's a good thing," he says.

Murphy also adds that, hand in hand with picturing your ultimate achievements, you also have to have a plan for making them happen. "It's good to visualize the steps you're going to take to make your fitness dreams come true," he says.

Use this daily meditation to help you lose weight and get in shape. Set aside five minutes each day for this simple yet effective exercise. It will keep you centered and help you focus both your mind and your body on your goals.

Find a quiet place, sit in a comfortable position, and close your eyes. Breathe deeply yet gently, inhaling through your nose, exhaling through your mouth. Concentrate on the feeling of your chest, lungs, and diaphragm expanding and contracting. Relax your entire body. After ten deep breaths, picture in your mind's eye a thinner, healthier version of yourself. Don't be judgmental about the way you look now; simply imagine your appearance once you've reached your fitness goals. Bask in the satisfaction that comes with your achievements. If your goals seem too overwhelming right now or you find them impossible to envision, imagine a point somewhere in the middle of the process. You can readjust this picture of yourself any way or as often as you like, so long as you think kind, uncritical thoughts about your body.

Pilates to the Core

In 2000, a landmark legal decision expanded the meaning of the term *Pilates*. Prior to this, Pilates meant only one thing: Your instructor went through coursework and a protracted internship sanctioned by the Pilates Institute in New York City. Pilates is now considered a generic phrase, much like yoga or kickboxing. This is good and bad news.

It's good news because Pilates is now more widely available. Almost every gym now offers Pilates classes; there are dozens of instructional videotapes, books, and magazine articles that were not obtainable under the old restrictions. It's bad news because now anyone can call herself a Pilates teacher—including someone with little or no training. This forces you to become a more savvy, educated consumer.

Before you set foot in a class or use your credit card to order the latest Pilates video, find out what kind of experience and expertise your instructor has. Having a Pilates certification is a plus, but they aren't all created equal. Ideally a certification should involve extensive study and internship under the tutelage of an experienced Pilates master. Many so-called certifications require little more than a weekend workshop and a passing grade on a written test that requires only the sketchiest knowledge.

THE PERFECT TRAVEL WORKOUT

Mary Duffy has traveled all over the world for business and pleasure yet still manages to stay fit and healthy. Some locations have presented more of a challenge than others as far as her fitness routine is concerned. For instance, though she loves to run and walk to keep in shape, she once spent two weeks in Morocco, where local custom frowned upon women dressed in exercise clothing appearing in public. "I had to work out in my hotel room the entire time," she remembers. Mary says that places off the beaten track where gyms are scarce, as well as traveling between radically different climates, can put a crimp in your exercise style if you don't come prepared and keep an open mind as far as workout possibilities are concerned. She always carries exercise tubing in her suitcase and often, on a moment's notice, improvises a workout routine like the one in this chapter.

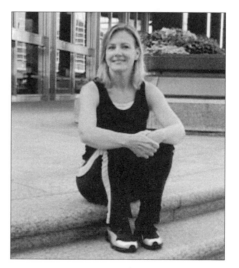

EXERCISES IN THIS CHAPTER

- Stair Walking
- Push-ups
- Squats

- Lunges
- Single-Leg Calf Raises
- Full Chair Dips
- Active Cat
- Shoulder Series
- Inner Thigh Taps
- Towel Abs

EQUIPMENT NEEDED

- Stairs
- A bath towel
- A sturdy, stable chair

ESTIMATED WORKOUT TIME

- 20–30 minutes, two to four times a week

My good friend Deb used to work for me as a group class coordinator, and she was a darned good one. She left to combine her two loves: fitness and travel. For the past couple of years she's been a fitness director for Norwegian Cruise Lines. "It is so great!" she gushed when I last spoke to her. "I get to travel all over the world, meet tons of people, and teach them all about getting in shape."

Deb's onboard weight-training seminars often draw over a hundred people, many of them older and many of them just learning for the first time about the importance of pumping iron. If you ever decide you want to take a fun-filled, workout-oriented vacation, I highly recommend booking a cruise with Deb. Be sure to tell her hello from me.

Unfortunately, it's not always so easy to stay in shape when you travel. There's rarely a Deb at your destination. You're more likely to wind up sitting in cramped quarters for hours, either on a plane or in a car, with so little opportunity to move around that you begin feeling like a stuffed veal roast. Healthy food is often a scarce commodity, too—one time on a six-hour flight to California I was served a bologna-and-mayonnaise sandwich on white bread with chips on the side. It was that or nothing. I chose nothing but was so famished by the time I got to my hotel that I almost didn't care what I ate. Toss jet lag, traffic jams, lack of sleep, and unfamiliar surroundings into the mix, and you've got a real shape-up challenge on your hands.

On-the-Road Rules

Keeping up with your fitness routine is hard enough when you're at home. On the road, it takes commitment, proactivity, and a bit of advance planning to make it work. In this section, I give you physical and logistical tips for exercising and eating well while you're on the road.

- **Make time for movement.** I like to get each trip off to a good start, so I try to do a workout or take a walk before I hop on a plane or get in the car for a long ride. I find this harder to do when I have an early departure, but I had one client, Amy, who was a frequent flyer known to drag her butt out of bed at three in the morning for a quick run on her treadmill before she headed to the airport. "It's not pleasant, but I figure I can always sleep on the plane," she rationalized. Amy said she felt more relaxed and less stressed when she ran before a flight, even if it was an abbreviated version of her normal mileage. As much as I agonize about getting up any earlier than I have to, I'm with Amy. You definitely feel better when you exercise before you travel. Remember when I said this takes commitment? I wasn't kidding!

  Once you're out the door, keep moving whenever you can. In airports and public places, avoid escalators and people movers, those slow-moving sidewalks that transport people from place to place like canned goods on a supermarket checkout conveyor belt. And keep moving as much as possible until it's time to depart; you'll have plenty of fanny-warming time once you're airborne or on the road.

  Wear walking or running shoes. You'll certainly be more comfortable, plus you're more likely to walk from place to place. When you reach your destination, if it's at all in the cards, do something mobile for at least twenty minutes rather than staying in the house or hotel.

And, in spite of what I've said about having limited chances to exercise en route, there are glimmers of progress. Some major airports are now home to state-of-the-art twenty-four-hour fitness centers. You can grab a quick workout for a reasonable fee while on a layover or if your flight is delayed. For a list of airports that have gyms, check out 24hourfitness.com. Sadly, drop-in fitness centers along major highways remain one of my unrealized million-dollar ideas.

- **Pack for a workout.** Always, always bring your basic workout gear with you even if you're only going for a short hop and even if you're pretty sure you won't be able to squeeze in a workout. You never know. If you're packed and ready to go, you're always prepared. If the opportunity arises, you'll kick yourself if you don't have the right shoes or clothes with you.

Remember, too, that the weather you're leaving behind is not necessarily the weather you're going toward. For this reason it helps to pack rain gear and clothing choices for both warmer and cooler possibilities. Make sure your rain gear is waterproof and not just water-resistant. Trust me when I tell you that there is a big difference between the two—a difference you don't want to discover during a rainy run through the middle of nowhere, as I did.

Bring emergency backup weight-training equipment, such as exercise bands or tubes (long, flat, narrow strips of rubber or rubber tubing that resemble the tubing found on blood pressure cuffs). A set of tubes or bands can cost as little as $10, but if you want to get fancy you can buy a rubber tubing mini-gym complete with a carrying case, video, and plastic bar for around a hundred bucks (Lifeline Gyms makes a good one).

I love tubing because you can mimic dozens of free-weight and machine strength-training exercises with them, yet they fit easily into a suitcase or purse. I like them much better than other travel weight alternatives, such as those water-filled dumbbells you see advertised in the back of travel magazines. My experience with them is that they're wobbly and leaky. I definitely don't recommend lugging around real steel dumbbells, as I once did—it wasn't worth the trouble, especially since I would have gotten more bang for the buck with a few ounces of exercise band.

For cardio, a jump rope or an exercise videotape make for excellent, inexpensive stowaways. I find hotel stairs are good for an impromptu fat-burning session, too. All three of these choices are suitable alternatives to your usual workout or run or if where you're staying doesn't have a decent workout room. Last year I found myself at an airport hotel in Toronto surrounded by nothing but runways and large-vehicle access roads. The so-called hotel gym was a total eighties flashback. For the two days I was there I did the travel workout you'll find in this chapter.

- **Plan ahead.** I try to stay in hotels that have gyms, so I either call ahead or suss out the situation on-line. However, be aware that what you're told or what's posted on the Net can sometimes be a wild exaggeration. I can't tell you how many hotels claim to have excellent fitness facilities and all you find when you get there is a battered Universal gym gathering dust in a corner or a lonely and dilapidated treadmill with an Out of Order sign taped to its console.

  That's why I always look for a backup workout location ahead of time. I either call the hotel and ask them what's in the neighborhood or check out the fitness center scene on-line. Healthclubs.com and healthclub.com are two good sources for this sort of information.

  If you can remember to do it, make all personal-training appointments and court reservations ahead of time. Fitness writer John Hanc uses traveling as an opportunity to try out new trainers and workouts. He says it's a great way to learn something new or try something different. But if you want to try to stick closely to your home base routine, bring a copy of your workout with you; even if you decide to hire a trainer, you can hand him a step-by-step guide of what you've been up to. (Or you can try an on-line trainer that "travels" with you. See World Wide Workout, page 266.)

- **Be creative.** On a business trip I took to Hong Kong a few years ago, I stayed in a five-star hotel with a pretty good fitness center.

Unfortunately, the handyman decided the gym was a great location to do all of the hotel's furniture repairs. I went in for a workout, and the glue and paint fumes were so strong they made me swoon. I complained to the manager, but he simply shrugged, informing me that this would be an ongoing project for several weeks. When I tried to find another gym in the area to use on a guest pass, I quickly discovered that most gyms in Hong Kong don't allow guests and that joining one, even for a short term, can cost thousands of dollars. Not to be deterred, I tried running in the streets, but Hong Kong packs over six million people onto an island two-thirds the size of Manhattan—the city streets are so crowded, it's tough to walk without bumping into other pedestrians, let alone zip along at the lightning speed of seven miles per hour. Finally, I settled on taking a taxi ride to the outer limits of the city to hike in one of the many national parks. On days I couldn't do that, I climbed stairs or exercised in my room. I finally made it home three weeks later having had an amazing experience I might otherwise have missed—a working knowledge of the Hong Kong park system—and my fitness level was more or less intact.

My point is, your usual workout may not be possible while you're traveling, so you may need to stretch your imagination along with your muscles. If your first choice doesn't pan out, try something else. If that doesn't fly, keep searching for a way to stay active. You can usually find something to do. Be ready to try new things, especially if that's all that is available.

- **Stay hydrated.** Air-conditioning in cars, planes, and hotels tends to shrivel you up like a century-old raisin. Not only does your skin dry out, so do your eyes and the mucous membranes in your nasal passages. Besides making you look and feel pasty and flaky, dryness predisposes you to infections. That's why it's so common to get sick shortly after you return from a trip.

    Bring water with you and keep sipping it as much as possible, especially during plane trips where you're exposed to recirculated air, the breathing equivalent of a musty old antique. Avoid alcohol, caffeine, and salt as well. All contribute to fluid loss and increase your chances of dehydration.

- **Watch what you eat.** The good and the bad of travel is being forced to eat virtually every meal at a restaurant. It's good because half the fun of going to new places is sampling local specialty dishes. It's bad because it can wreak havoc on your body fat percentage.

When dining out, think calorie budget. Watch out for dish descriptions peppered with cooking terms: *Sautéed* means pan-fried in butter, *tempura* means batter-coated and fried, *au gratin* means drenched in cheese sauce. Other terms to beware of: *fried, deep-fried, pan-fried, crispy, braised, creamed, hollandaise, escalloped.* Terms that signal healthy choices: *steamed, broiled* (a little butter or oil is okay), *"in its own juice," garden-fresh, roasted, lemon,* and *wine.*

Order sauces, dressings, and gravies on the side. Ask your waiter how dishes are prepared, and perhaps he can steer you toward the lightest choices on the menu. Also request that he not place butter or other fattening fare on the table.

If you have your heart set on deep-fried catfish or a crème brûlée, consider eating half and doggy-bagging the rest, or share with your dining partners. You can also save calories by ordering à la carte. This way you don't feel obliged to eat massive amounts of food simply because you paid for it.

But as fattening as hotel and restaurant meals can be, the meals you eat getting to your destination are the worst diet saboteurs on the planet. I already told you about being served a bologna sandwich on a flight. And how many times have you driven into a highway rest stop where you have a choice between McDonald's, Burger King, and the vending machine?

Try to avoid life in the fast-food lane at all costs, but if you can't, at least order wisely. I don't need to tell you that anything that contains the words *big, jumbo, double,* or *special sauce* in the menu description is probably not the best thing for your waistline or arteries. Ironically, sometimes seemingly healthier fare such as chicken, fish, and vegetarian items turn out to be the highest-fat, most calorie-laden selections on the menu. For example, a Schlotzsky's Western Vegetarian Sandwich weighs in at 1,261 calories and packs a whopping sixty-one grams of fat per serving. (Your recommended total daily intake of fat should only be around sixty-five grams!) Use common sense; stick to basic sandwiches, or split a meal with someone else. (See the sidebar "The Fittest (and Fattest) Fast Foods" on page 263 for the skinny on which fast foods are the least and most fattening.)

Here's a great tip for when you fly: Many airlines offer special healthy meals you can request in advance. You can often order anything from kosher to vegetarian to low-fat to nondairy. In addition to containing healthier ingredients, they are often fresher and tastier because they are individually prepared.

And to be fair, most airlines serve something more sensible than bologna these days, and many roadside fast-food joints now offer at least a few lighter meals—but you do need to be extremely diligent when seeking out healthier foods when you travel. I usually carry along my own snacks because it gives me total control over what I'm eating and takes away all my excuses to eat unwisely.

- **Don't cause unnecessary pain.** Traveling can be a pain in the neck. Literally. My client Amy used to come home from business trips with a sore neck from slinging her bag around her neck as she dashed to catch her flight. She often had to skip training sessions until the pain went away. She finally bought one of those bags on wheels you can roll along behind you. Problem solved.

  Like Amy, consider investing in luggage that's more ergonomic. Most luggage companies make good lines specially designed for those with neck, back, elbow, and shoulder problems. Always practice good lifting mechanics as well; bend at the knees to pick up something heavy, as opposed to bending at the waist, which turns your back into a lightning rod for injuries. When you carry something in your hand, don't allow your arm to hang straight down; keep a slight bend in your elbow to limit stress on your delicate elbow and shoulder joints. If you travel with a backpack, don't overload it, and choose one that has plenty of back and shoulder padding, a hip strap to help take some of the weight off your back and shoulders, and a sternum strap that buckles across the chest to take pressure off the shoulders and neck. Eastpak and Arc'teryx are two backpack companies I've always had good luck with, but they are by no means the only ones that make comfortable travel packs. I recently bought my husband a "lap sack," a specially designed backpack for transporting your laptop computer. It's so well designed and comfortable, I've stolen it from him (as I do with all the good presents I buy him).

If you're prone to back pain, taking frequent stretch breaks is a must. You can also place a rolled-up small towel or pillow behind the small of your back. When driving, use cruise control and stretch every opportunity you get. When you're stopped at red lights, contract and relax your buttocks until the light changes. Believe it or not, this helps relieve back fatigue, plus it's a subtle enough move not to attract any attention from other drivers. You probably can't get away with it in the close quarters of coach class on a plane, though.

- **Adjust your expectations.** When all is said and done, while you're on the road you may not be able to work out at the same level you do at home. As soon as you return, pick up your routine where you left off. Though traveling can be disruptive to your workout schedule, it does not have to be devastating. I always tell clients to aim to maintain some minimums, and not to be too hard on themselves if their fitness level takes a small dip. Do what you can, but don't skip *everything* just because you don't have time to do it all. A little something is better than a lot of nothing.

The Perfect Travel Exercises

This is the one routine in the book I don't think you'll be using on a regular basis, though there really isn't any reason why you can't. It certainly contains all of the elements you need to get your body in shape.

Assuming you use this workout only as an occasional fallback when you aren't able to do your normal routine, you won't make progress per se. But if you decide to use it consistently as a home routine if you don't have any equipment, I recommend doing it two to four times a week. Do one to three sets of all of the exercises unless otherwise noted; do eight to fifteen reps per set, again unless otherwise noted. You'll see progress in the form of increased stamina and a more toned body (especially the lower body) in about one month.

If you need to make things more challenging, you can add rubber tubing, as I've suggested in the harder versions of some of the exercises. As an alternative, you can hold two equally weighted objects, but this requires some creativity. You can try two phone books, bookends, or full-size shampoo bottles. Personally, I think you'll find the exercise bands a more comfortable, natural way to challenge yourself.

■ STAIR WALKING

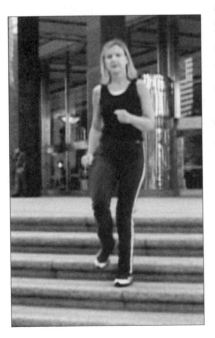

Muscles Worked: This is an awesomely effective cardio and calorie-burning exercise. It tones your buttocks, thighs, and calves. It's a great alternative if you don't have access to a decent gym or if there isn't a good place to walk or run. To start, do three to ten sets of stairs. Be careful not to overdo it; walking stairs, especially down the stairs, can cause extreme soreness.

Joint Cautions: Lower back; strong caution for knees.

Walking Up: Walk up the stairs, taking them one at a time. Make sure you set your entire foot on each stair. Pump your arms vigorously; use them to help you power your movement. Walk up eight to ten flights.

Walking Down: Once you have reached the top of the last flight, turn around and walk down to your starting point. Stay up on your toes and move carefully, holding on to the banister if you need help with balance. Move quickly but stay in control.

Things to Think About:

- When walking upstairs, lean slightly forward from the hips to take pressure off your lower back.
- Always set your entire foot on each stair; this will protect your knees and ankles and provide maximum stability.

Variations:

- **EASIER:** Hold on to the banister when walking upstairs. Support yourself only as much as you need to.
- **HARDER:** Jog up the stairs. Or, every other flight, take the stairs two at a time, always being careful to land with your entire foot on the step.

■ PUSH-UPS

Muscles Worked: An excellent exercise for your chest muscles that also works your shoulders, triceps, and abdominals.

Joint Cautions: Shoulders, elbows, lower back.

Starting Position: Lie on your stomach with your legs out straight, feet a few inches apart. Bend your elbows and place your palms on the floor slightly to the side and in front

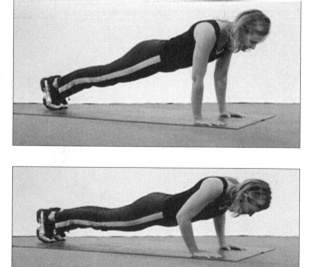

of your shoulders. Straighten your arms and press your body upward so that your arms are nearly straight and you're balanced on your palms and the underside of your toes. Tuck your chin a few inches toward your chest so that your forehead faces the floor. Pull your abdominal muscles inward.

Exercise: Bend your elbows to lower your body. When your elbows are level with your shoulders, press back up to the start.

Things to think about:

- Keep your entire back, including your buttocks, straight and level; even when you move, imagine balancing something delicate on top of your back that you don't want to fall off and break. You'll feel the backs of your arms, center of your shoulders, and center of your chest working, especially as you straighten your arms.
- Think of initiating the movement by pressing your palms down into the floor to lift your body upward.
- Avoid bending your elbows below shoulder level; this puts excess strain on the shoulders and rotator cuff.

Variations:

- **EASIER:** Do a modified push-up: Rather than holding your body straight out, bend your knees so that you're balanced on the tops of your thighs just above your knees. If this is still too challenging, try a wall push-up, as described on pages 51–52.
- **HARDER:** Hold the bottom part of the movement for a count of two before pushing up to the start.

■ SQUATS

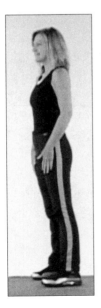 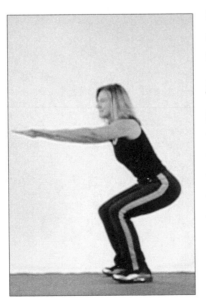

Muscles Worked: One of the best exercises you can do to strengthen and tone the buttocks and thighs.

Joint Cautions: Knees, lower back.

Starting Position: Place your hands on the tops of your thighs and stand with your feet hip width apart, with your weight slightly back on your heels. Pull your abdominals in and stand up tall with square shoulders.

Exercise: Bend your knees to lower your body. You can extend your arms up in front of your shoulders if you feel that helps you balance. Once your thighs are parallel to the floor, stand back up to the starting position.

Things to Think About:

- Imagine you are sitting down into a chair that is directly behind you as you lower yourself. You'll feel the muscles in the front of your thighs contracting when you stand back up to the start; some people also feel their buttocks muscles working.
- How far you lower yourself depends on your flexibility. You may only be able to bend your knees a few inches before your upper body folds too far forward, or you may be able to keep your back straight until your thighs are parallel to the floor. Just don't allow your knees to move forward of your toes.
- When you stand up, don't fully straighten or lock your knees.

Variations:

- **EASIER:** Place a chair behind you and let your butt touch lightly on the seat before standing back up.
- **HARDER:** Stand on the center of an exercise band with an end in each hand. Bend your elbows and hold your hands up near your shoulders to create tension in the band. Do the exercise using the same form as the basic version; the band will create resistance as you stand back up to the starting position.

■ LUNGES

Muscles Worked: A focused buttocks and thigh toner.

Joint Cautions: Lower back, knees.

Starting Position: Stand with your feet straddled a stride's length apart and your weight slightly forward on your right foot. Place your hands on your hips, pull your abdominals in, and stand up tall with square shoulders.

Exercise: Bend both knees until your right knee is parallel to the floor and your left is perpendicular to it; at this point your left heel will be

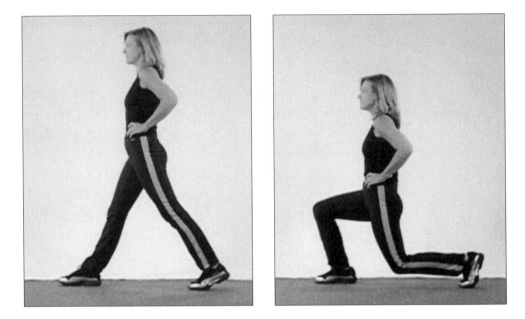

lifted off the floor. Press off the ball of your right foot to stand back up. Complete all reps on the right side and then repeat with your left leg in front.

Things to Think About:
- You'll feel a strong contraction in the front of your thighs as you bend your knees, and a stretch through the back of your thighs (and possibly your inner thighs) as you step forward.
- Imagine you are stepping over a crack on the sidewalk as you step forward.
- Don't let your front knee travel in front of your toes.

Variations:
- **EASIER:** Hold on to a sturdy object for support and balance.
- **HARDER:** Stand in the starting position, with the center of an exercise band underneath your forward foot and an end wrapped in each hand. Do the same basic exercise; the band will provide resistance as you stand back up.

■ SINGLE-LEG CALF RAISES

Muscles Worked: Isolates your calf muscles.

Joint Cautions: Slight ankle caution.

Starting Position: Stand tall with your feet together and hold on to a sturdy object with one hand for support. Lift your right foot off the floor and wrap it around behind your left ankle so it is out of the way.

Exercise: Pressing through your toes and the ball of your foot, lift your left heel off the floor as high as you can. Hold a moment and then lower to the start. Complete the set and repeat with your right leg.

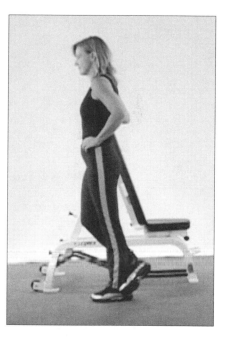

Things to Think About:
• Press straight upward without allowing your ankle to wobble inward or outward. You'll feel a strong pull through the entire length of your calves as you rise and a stretch as you lower.

Variations:
• EASIER: Rather than lifting your heel up as high as you can, press upward only a few inches.
• HARDER: Sit on the floor with your legs out in front of you, with one foot raised a few inches off the floor, an exercise band securely wrapped around the instep and an end of the band held in each hand. Press your toe forward to create resistance in the band and then press your heel forward. Or you can do the basic version of this exercise with your heels hanging off the edge of a step so that when you lower, your heels go past the starting point and you feel a stretch through your calves.

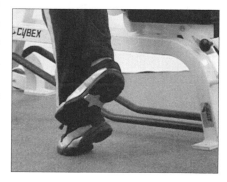

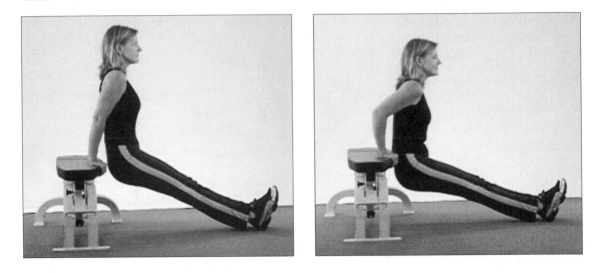

■ FULL CHAIR DIPS

Muscles Worked: Your triceps, chest, and shoulder muscles.

Joint Cautions: Shoulders, rotator cuff.

Starting Position: Sit on the edge of a stable chair with your hands on either side of you gripping the underside of the seat. Straighten your legs out in front of you with your heels on the floor, toes up. Slide your butt off the chair so that it's hovering an inch or two forward of the chair seat. Pull your belly button in toward your spine and keep your torso straight.

Exercise: Bend your elbows and lower your body toward the floor. When your upper arms are parallel to the floor or slightly above, press back up to the starting position.

Things to Think About:
• In the starting position you should look like you're sitting in an imaginary lounge chair whose front is tilted all the way to the floor. You'll feel a strong pull through the backs of your upper arms, the center of your shoulders, and possibly the edges of your chest as you straighten your arms.

- Make sure you are lowering yourself by bending your elbows rather than by shifting your shoulders forward and back.
- Keep your shoulders down and relaxed, and avoid lowering your upper arms below parallel.

Variations:

- **EASIER:** Do the Basic Triceps Dip as described in "The Perfect Beginner Workout" on page 58.
- **HARDER:** Keeping your legs straight, place your heels up on a chair or another raised surface.

■ ACTIVE CAT

Muscles Worked: This exercise feels great because, in addition to strengthening the lower back and hip and thigh muscles, it's also an excellent stretch for the lower back, abs, hips, and thighs.

Joint Cautions: Mild caution for lower back. May actually help those with lower back issues.

Starting Position: Get down on your hands and knees on a towel. Gently pull your belly button in toward your spine. Inhale deeply through your nose and tuck your right knee and your head in toward your chest.

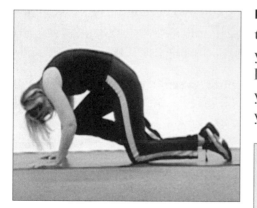

Exercise: Exhale slowly and deeply through your mouth as you stretch your right leg up and out behind you, lengthening your spine and lifting your head up. Complete all reps with your right leg and then with your left.

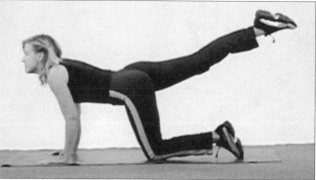

Things to Think About:

- As the name implies, this exercise mimics a cat stretching. You'll feel your lower back muscles contract moderately as you fold inward and outward. You'll also feel a stretch through the entire length of your spine and leg as you fully extend.
- In the starting position your lower back should not hunch upward or sag downward.
- You don't need to overdo the fully extended position of this exercise.

Variations:

- **EASIER:** Eliminate the upper-body movement.
- **HARDER:** In the fully extended position, lower your leg toward the floor three times before moving into the next repetition; this will increase the hip and thigh involvement.

▇ SHOULDER SERIES

Muscles Worked: An excellent shoulder-toning series.

Joint Cautions: Mild shoulder and rotator cuff caution.

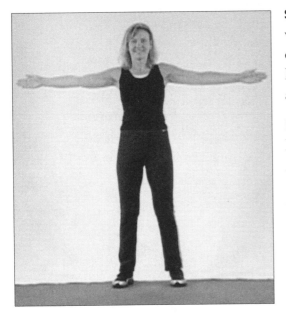

Starting Position: Stand tall with your feet hip width apart and your arms extended up and out to the sides, your palms facing forward. Keep your chest lifted, your shoulders relaxed and down, and your abs pulled inward.

Exercise: Slowly circle your arms forward, keeping the circles small and well formed. After ten circles, reverse the direction. Then do ten circles forward and back with your palms facing down and, after that, with your palms facing upward.

Things to Think About:

- Imagine your fingertips are drawing a circle on the walls about the size of a salad bowl.

You will feel a strong pull through your shoulders that will gradually grow stronger as you continue the exercise.

- Focus on extending your arms to maximum length while staying relaxed.

Variations:
- **EASIER:** Take a break after every set of circles.
- **HARDER:** Stand on one end of the band while holding the other end in one hand. Raise your arm up and out to the side until you feel sufficient resistance created in the band and then slowly lower to the starting position.

■ INNER THIGH TAPS

Muscles Worked: Besides working your inner thighs, this exercise helps develop a sense of coordination.

Joint Cautions: None.

Starting Position: Lie on your left side with your head resting on your outstretched arm and your abs pulled inward; place your right palm on the floor in front of you for support. Straighten your legs out a few inches in front of you so that your right hip is stacked directly on top of your left hip. Hold your right leg up a few inches in the air with your toe softly pointed and your knee turned up toward the ceiling.

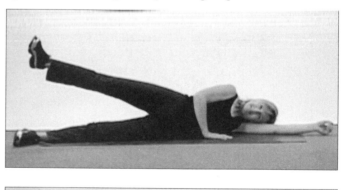

Exercise: Lift your left leg upward and quickly tap your heels together ten times. This is one repetition. Lower your left leg between repetitions.

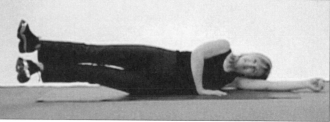

Things to Think About:

- This exercise may feel awkward when you first try it. You may have trouble tapping your heels or staying in balance. That's okay. You'll get more precise and less awkward each time you do the exercise.
- You'll feel a contraction through the inner thigh of your bottom leg the entire time you're tapping.

Variations:

- **EASIER:** Bend both of your knees slightly; this will make it easier to control the movement.
- **HARDER:** Tie a band in a tight circle around your ankles. Lift your top leg up a few inches until you create resistance in the band and then slowly lower to the start.

■ TOWEL ABS

Muscles Worked: This exercise targets your abdominal muscles.

Joint Cautions: None. In fact, this is a good alternative if you often experience neck or back pain when working your abs.

Starting Position: Place a large bath towel on the floor and lie on your back on top of it so that your head is near one end. Bend your knees and place your feet flat on the floor. Grab a corner of the towel with each hand. Tip your chin back slightly and pull your abs inward.

Exercise: Curl your head, neck, and shoulders up and forward off the floor, pulling up on the towel to assist you. Hold a moment and then lower to the starting position.

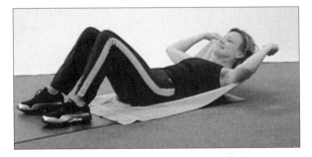 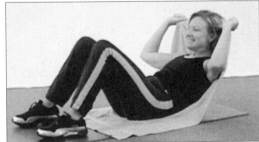

Things to Think About:

- This exercise mimics an Ab Roller but does a better job working the abs. The towel helps support your neck so that you can focus on working your ab muscles. You'll feel your ab muscles working the hardest as you reach the top of the movement and hold it a moment.
- Exhale through your mouth as you lift; inhale through your nose as you lower.
- Avoid yanking upward too forcefully on the towel.

Variations:

- EASIER: Use the towel more to assist your upward movement.
- HARDER: As you lift up, twist to the side. Alternate sides each rep.

The Fittest (and Fattest) Fast Foods

Obviously, a fast-food joint is not an optimal place to dine if you're minding calories and fat, but sometimes you gotta do what you gotta do. For navigating your way through the various fat and calorie contents of popular fast-food selections, I offer you the following guidelines. As you can see, it's easier to make better selections in some places than in others. In my opinion, Burger King is the toughest place to make a healthy choice.

This chart is meant as a representative list of choices, and I haven't necessarily given you the highest- or lowest-calorie options from each menu. Also, notice that some of the lower-calorie choices aren't exactly low in fat, and vice versa.

Fast Food	Best Choices	Fat grams/% of calories from fat	Calories	Worst Choices	Fat grams/% of calories from fat	Calories
McDonald's	Hamburger	9g/30%	270	Big Xtra w/Cheese	55g/61%	810
	Grilled Chicken Caesar Salad w/fat free vinaigrette, no croutons	2.5g/23%	100	Crispy Chicken Deluxe	24g/40%	550

Fast Food	Best Choices	Fat grams/% of calories from fat	Calories	Worst Choices	Fat grams/% of calories from fat	Calories
McDonald's (Cont.)	Fruit and Yogurt Parfait, no Granola	4g/13%	260	Nestle Crunch® McFlurry	24g/34%	630
Burger King	Hamburger	15g/42%	320	Double Whopper w/Cheese	67g/60%	1010
	Chicken Tenders, 4 pieces, no sauce	11g/55%	180	Chicken Sandwich	43g/55%	710
	Small fries	13g/47%	250	Large Onion Rings	30g/45%	600
Kentucky Fried Chicken	Tender Roast Chicken w/o skin	2.4g/32%	67	Extra Tasty Crispy Breast	28g/54%	470
	Value BBQ Chicken Sandwich	8g/28%	256	Chunky Chicken Pot Pie	42g/49%	770
	Mashed Potatoes w/ Gravy (Side)	6g/45%	120	Potato Salad	14g/53%	240
Wendy's	Jr. Hamburger	10g/33%	270	Big Bacon Classic	30g/47%	580
	Small Chili, no toppings	7g/30%	210	Chili & Cheese Potato	24g/35%	630
	Grilled Chicken Salad, Fat Free French dressing	9g/34%	235	Pita Chicken Caesar	18g/33%	490
Arby's	Arby-Q®	15g/36%	380	Big Montana®	40g/50%	720
	Lt. Grilled Chicken Salad, Buttermilk Ranch Dressing Reduced Cal.	4g/15%	240	Roast Chicken Panini	38g/40%	855
	Potato Pancakes	14g/57%	220	Deluxe Baked Potato	31g/46%	610
Taco Bell	Taco	10g/50%	180	Taco Salad, Salsa	52g/55%	850

Fast Food	Best Choices	Fat grams/% of calories from fat	Calories	Worst Choices	Fat grams/% of calories from fat	Calories
Taco Bell (cont.)	Fiesta Chicken Gordita	10g/35%	260	Chicken Supreme Fajita Wrap	26g/45%	520
	Mexican Rice	9g/43%	190	Nacho Bellgrande	39g/46%	770
Sample pizza selections	1 slice pizza (typical parlor pie, average size slices)	12.5g/38%	300	1 slice The Big New Yorker Sausage Pizza	33g/54%	550

Training Travel

Vacation doesn't have to mean two weeks vegetating by a pool or cruising all-you-can-eat buffets. An invigorating and satisfying alternative is to plan an active vacation, or at least one that's partially oriented toward being healthy. You feel so much better when you come home! Here are three of my favorite sources for active vacations.

- **Backroads:** This travel organization offers biking, walking, hiking, and multi-sport vacations all over North America, Europe, Asia, the Pacific, South America, and Africa. It is the number one active travel agency in the world. I've never taken one of their tours, but many of my friends and clients have; I hear good things. Backroads offers all types of trips for all budgets and tastes, including first-class hotel accommodations, gourmet dining, van-trailer support, and pro-fessional trip leaders. They have two- to fifteen-day inn and camping trips for all ages and abilities (backroads.com).

- **Explore Britain Walking Holidays:** Formerly the English Wanderer tour group, this organization offers self-guided tours from inn to inn throughout the British Isles. They give you maps and descriptions of how to get from point A to point B, and you go on your own without a guide. It's really not as hard as it sounds, plus they transport your luggage from place to place and provide most of your meals. My husband and I did a tour along the south coast of Wales, where the ocean is juxtaposed with farmland and thousand-year-old castles. It was the best vacation we ever took (xplorebritain.com).

- **European Ramblers Association (ERA):** Founded in 1969, the European Ramblers Association is a federation, currently based in Germany, of fifty-six walking organizations from twenty-seven European countries. Contact them for both guided and self-guided European walking vacations and maps of European footpaths. My husband and I took one of their self-guided inn-to-inn tours of the French wine country and had a spectacular time. The cost was reasonable as well (gorp.com).

World Wide Workout

It used to be that traveling with a personal trainer was reserved for the rich and famous. Now your trainer can follow you around the world for less than $30 a month. All you need is Internet access and a membership to an on-line personal training service.

I never used to be a big fan of on-line trainers, but my experience on both sides of the fence—as a trainer and as a client—is that they are not without merit. Granted, they will never take the place of a live trainer standing over you screaming "One more rep!" but the good ones are perfect for health-conscious globe-trotters who crave continuity in their workouts. They offer expert advice at a bargain price and tons of scheduling flexibility.

When looking for a good on-line trainer, follow the same guidelines as you would when looking for a good flesh-and-blood trainer. Choose a service that offers you a one-to-one relationship with an individual as opposed to a computer or a pool of nameless, faceless trainers; look for top-drawer credentials such as certification, fitness-related college degrees, and many years of experience; opt for a service that offers valuable extras such as quick response time, e-mail workout reminders, feedback forms, a workout calendar, an exercise library, and progress charts. A good one: myfitnessexpert.com.

INDEX

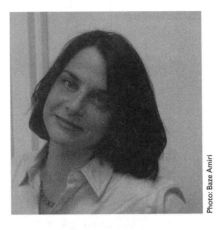

ABOUT THE AUTHOR

Liz Neporent has been in the business of helping people get in shape for more than fifteen years. She is currently the creative director for Plus One Health Management, a fitness consulting company in New York City. Her job is to make sure fitness center members for more than a twenty-five clubs in hotels and corporations throughout the country are happy, motivated, and exercising on a regular basis.

Liz holds a master's degree in exercise physiology and is certified by the American Council on Exercise, the American College of Sports Medicine, the National Strength and Conditioning Association, and the National Academy of Sports Medicine. She is on the board of the American Council on Exercise and the advisory board for several publications, including Fitness magazine.

Liz is coauthor of *Buns of Steel: Total-Body Workout, Abs of Steel,* and *Weight Training for Dummies.* She is also author of *Fitness Walking for Dummies* and writes a regular column, "Fit by Friday," for iVillage.com. Additionally, she is a regular contributor to various publications including the *New York Times, Newsday, Fitness* magazine, *Shape, Family Circle,* and others. She appears regularly on TV and radio as an authority on fitness and exercise.

Liz is an avid runner and has competed in more than two dozen marathons and ultramarathons. She is also devoted to sports climbing, Pilates, hiking, jump rope, and weight training. She lives in New York City where she walks to work and takes additional daily walks with her husband, Jay Shafran, and her greyhound, Zoomer.